Pr

unforgotten
CHILDREN

This book will bring hope and healing from the pain and loss of miscarriage to a multitude of women. Kristie's trust in the Lord, in all circumstances, is evident and brings hope and reality to the reader as she shares her own loss of two children to miscarriage. This book is a must-read for all women who have shared that same heartache.

—Cathy Goggin

I'm speechless... you have captured the heart of every grieving mother in your book! You have explained so fluently the things that I wish I could have expressed throughout my healing journey.

—Kari Fuhrman

Your experience in the hospital sadly has been and will be repeated over and over. Your story will encourage mothers that have miscarried to open their hearts to others that have been silenced by pain and rejection. Those who read this will be impacted by the depth of emotion and be motivated to grow from the past that binds. There is freedom in Jesus. He wants to heal, not only our bodies but our thoughts and feelings. Be ye transformed by the renewing of your mind (Romans 12:2).

—Barbara Christiansen

One cannot read this and not feel gripped even in the slightest way. I urge you, if you come from this story completely untouched, please, check your pulse.

—Martha C. Gehbauer

unforgotten CHILDREN

unforgotten CHILDREN

A Testimony of God's Healing through Miscarriage

KRISTIE VERRET

TATE PUBLISHING *&* *Enterprises*

Published by Tate Publishing & Enterprises, LLC
127 E. Trade Center Terrace | Mustang, Oklahoma 73064 USA
1.888.361.9473 | www.tatepublishing.com

Tate Publishing is committed to excellence in the publishing industry. The company reflects the philosophy established by the founders, based on Psalm 68:11,
"The Lord gave the word and great was the company of those who published it."

Book design copyright © 2009 by Tate Publishing, LLC. All rights reserved.
Cover design by Kandi Evans
Interior design by Joey Garrett

Published in the United States of America

ISBN: 978-1-60799-937-9
1. Biography & Autobiography / Personal Memoirs
2. Health & Fitness / Pregnancy & Childbirth
09.09.01

DEDICATION

I would like to dedicate this book to my beautiful children, whose beauty in spirit far outweighs the wonders of this world.

"This you see, and think of me not unkind. For tho' your face I seldom see, you are ever on my mind. Love A.J.B." (by Alice Bellamore Theriot)

ACKNOWLEDGMENTS

To my Lord: I would like to offer thanks to you, Lord, for your almighty power. Through me, you have spoken where there was no voice. I give this book to you to use for your own glory. I offer my deepest gratitude to you, my Lord and Savior Jesus Christ. You have shown me, by example, what true love and family really are. I sincerely am grateful to you, Holy Spirit, for interpreting for me, and I know the blessings in my life overflow every day in good times and bad because of your unfailing love and devotion to me.

To my husband: Jack, you are my rock. I love you from the depths of my soul, for now and all the forevers. I thank God that you were the one he chose for me. Cheers to you for who you are not only in Christ but also for who you are as a husband, father, and character example for all who know you.

To my family: I would also like to recognize Mr. Jack and Mrs. Mary. You have been a life-changing factor for me, many years, and I thank you for it. You haven't been given the thanks you deserve, so I thank you now.

To my friends: Ronda, anyone who knows me knows my genuine love for you and my gratitude that God brought you into my life. God used you as a means of healing my spirit in a way that no one else could offer. You and I are forever connected through Sammi. My heart has etched an extraordinary place for you forever. Mrs. Gayle, I want to describe all of what you mean to me, but how can I? Your presence in my life has been so designed by God, and I am grateful for you being a part of it. You are not only a mentor to me but also a dear friend. Thank you for your calming influence! I want to offer also a special thanks to Stacie. Our hearts are forever bonded through Sammi. I want to recognize St. John's Lutheran Church (pastors and members) and Autumn Ridge Church (HOPE Ministries) for their constant attention to our needs and feelings during such a difficult time. We have not forgotten God's blessings to us through you.

The many others: I also want to give my sincerest appreciation to all the people who have contacted me during the time of my loss and in response to my speaking out about this experience. Your positive cards and encouragements have been crucial in my journey, and I thank you.

CHAPTER ONE

When I walked into the sanctuary that chilly Wednesday morning, my eyes immediately went to the altar. There was an oval-shaped wicker basket in the center of the table, surrounded by twelve unlit candles and twelve various colored roses. Each candle and rose stood as a symbol for twelve babies gone to heaven. I was only one of the five mothers who had come to honor her lost babies. Whether it was miscarriage, stillbirth, or early infant loss, we were all there for the same reason: to bury the sorrow of losing our babies and to accept God's healing in its place. As I walked toward my seat, carrying a handful of gifts for the other mothers, straight away, I felt my initial peace swiftly become nervousness.

I looked down at the two faceless baby dolls in my arms, which were intended to be representations of my two miscarried children, and I wondered, *How can I fully let them go?* One of the difficulties of my first miscarriage was the lack of something to hold on to; circumstances do not always allow for a burial. These dolls were meant to give me something that I could symbolically release. During my time with them, I was supposed to focus on remembering my children, but I wasn't ready to face letting go. Suddenly, I felt a twinge of guilt for spending such little time with the dolls and so much time avoiding them. This guilt truly embodied the beginning of my miscarriage journey.

I remember how adamantly I avoided looking at the truth about my first pregnancy loss. My poor Elizabeth was born to heaven in May of 2004, but for over three years, I refused to let anyone know about her short life and what she meant to us. Although God gave us every indication of her existence, I allowed the world to talk me out of acknowledging her outside of my own home. *I should have been more courageous,* I thought. *No,* I had to push that voice of regret aside. I would have no time to think of my mistakes. This memorial was meant to contribute to my healing; self-condemnation was to be left behind.

I gave my gifts to the director for her to place out of sight until the end of the ceremony. As I glanced over the order of service sheet, I noticed that my name was first on the list of mothers to share tributes. I had chosen to write a letter to honor my girls. Writing had always been my tool for healing. I smiled and waved at the other mothers as they arrived, and we all tried to pretend we weren't nearly as nervous as we each secretly felt. We listened as the director began by reading the first verse, "I will give them—within the walls of my house—a memorial and a name far greater than sons and daughters could give. For the name I give them is an everlasting one. It will never disappear!" (Isaiah 56:5).

I anxiously squeezed my fingers together while trying to withhold heavy tears from bursting forth, and

I shivered nervously. I could feel myself beginning to sweat. The first song that played was Elizabeth's song. I closed my eyes in an attempt to withstand the immense grief that was gradually swelling up inside me. I felt a tear run down my cheek, and I immediately grabbed a tissue in an attempt to quickly hide my tears. I am not sure why I felt so fearful of crying that day, but for some reason, I dreaded those tears.

Though the opening prayers had somewhat relieved my anxieties, the uneasiness caused by my fears promptly returned. The director read a few more scriptures.

> "For I know the plans I have for you," says the Lord. "They are plans for good and not for disaster, to give you a future and a hope. In those days when you pray, I will listen. If you look for me wholeheartedly, you will find me. I will be found by you," says the Lord. "I will end your captivity and restore your fortunes. I will gather you out of the nations where I sent you and will bring you home again to your own land."
>
> Jeremiah 29:11–14

> "But forget all that—it is nothing compared to what I am going to do. For I am about to do something new. See, I have already begun! Do you not see it? I will make a pathway through the wilderness. I will create rivers in the dry wasteland."
>
> Isaiah 43:18–19

Then it was my turn to speak. My hands shook as I grabbed the back of the pew in front of me to steady myself. I literally felt faint. *Don't pass out; don't pass out!* I silently begged in a quick prayer. I walked slowly to the altar, carrying my baby dolls and my letter.

When I arrived at the altar, the basket seemed so empty, utterly symbolic of my womb. I was the last mom in the group to lose her babies and the first to let them go. Ever so gently, I placed my dolls inside the basket. I rested my hand on their little white dresses and acknowledged to God my offering in a single-word prayer, "There." I lit the candle near Elizabeth's name, and then I lit Samantha's candle. I stood by the altar and began to read my letter. I nervously swayed my weight from one foot to the other, exposing my soul to these women once again. My words flowed freely, and my memory was forever imprinted with the scent of vanilla as it drifted from my children's candles.

CHAPTER TWO

Sometime, early in the year 2004, I had a very strange experience. Allie was nine months old, and Jack and I were longing for another baby to join our family. During the beginning of that year, I woke up in the middle of the night. I opened my eyes and looked over at my daughter's crib in our bedroom. Remarkably, she was awake. I saw her sitting up in her crib, looking at me. I sat up abruptly, thinking, *What kind of a mother are you? You didn't know she was awake?* I looked over at my husband to discover if he was awake, and on his arm, I saw Allie sleeping. I almost didn't believe it. I looked back at her crib, and in my state of confusion, I saw that she wasn't there. She had never even been to bed in her crib. I thought, *Did I just imagine that?* I was tired and disregarded it.

The following night, I awoke again and saw my daughter sitting underneath the desk in our room. Once more, I sat up abruptly, this time thinking, *Oh no! The outlet!* I glanced over to see where Jack was, and he was sleeping soundly with Allie on his chest. I fell back on the pillow, wondering if I was actually losing my mind. The next morning, I intentionally looked under the desk, and there were boxes piled there to hide the outlet, leaving no room for a baby to have even sat there. Unsure whether or not I was losing my mind, I decided not to mention it.

On the third night, I awoke again but did not sit up quickly. I just opened my eyes and noticed something sitting at my feet. When I looked down, I saw my daughter on the edge of the bed. There she sat, just looking at me. I kept my eyes on her for a few seconds to be sure that I was really seeing her, and as I turned my head toward my husband, I saw Allie asleep in between us. I looked back at my feet, and she wasn't there. *What is this? Is this a dream, a vision? What could this mean?* I wondered. I didn't tell anyone about what I saw because I didn't want anyone to think I was losing my mind. In fact, I wasn't entirely sure that I wasn't losing my mind. *Besides, I was probably just dreaming in that half-awake state*, I told myself.

In May, Allie turned one year old. Later that month, I began having a really severe period. I thought, *This is to be expected since I've missed several of my cycles.* Taking into consideration that irregular periods were normal for me, we thought nothing of it. Jack took me to his mom's house because I could barely walk from the severity of the cramping and I needed help with Allie.

Just before he left for work, I went to the bathroom, and this odd thing happened. I was not bleeding. I sat down, and something fell out of me. I stood up, surprised and horrified, and I saw this little piece of bean-shaped tissue in the toilet. I wasn't sure what to think. I called down the hall for Jack. I asked him to look and to see what he thought of the apparent flesh, and he said, "I don't know; maybe you should call the doctor."

The first doctor said that I had probably miscarried but if I had already passed "it" then the pregnancy test would show negative. I felt a numb sensation wash over my heart. It was a familiar feeling, the same reaction I had when my uncle told me that my mother died. I fell utterly into a state of shock. My next reaction was outright denial. *No, I couldn't be pregnant. I would have known. How could this be?*

I went to a local family doctor on Monday when they opened, and they took some blood work. The test said I was pregnant. I faxed the results to my gynecologist, who was located out of town (considering we had recently moved). The nurse called me and said, "You are not pregnant, and if you think you are, then you need to see a psychiatrist." I was completely devastated. I didn't know how to feel. Did I just lose a baby or not? If not, then what just fell out of my body? I was too afraid and embarrassed to contact yet another doctor.

I spent the next few months trying to overlook the whole experience, acting as if nothing had happened, but for some reason I couldn't forget. Finally, a few humiliated and confused months later, I talked to a third doctor. He said it was too late now but that the matter could have been resolved easily with an ultrasound. I didn't want to hear any more opinions on the subject. I was hurt, distraught, and confused. I didn't need people telling me that I was crazy.

Because I could not confirm the pregnancy, I never spoke with anyone else about it. I worried that others wouldn't believe me or worse yet, that I would be seen as obsessive or delusional. *It doesn't matter to anyone anyway, right?* I told myself. My husband didn't want to upset me, so he didn't mention it either. It somehow just became a secret, an unofficial forbidden subject.

One morning several weeks later, my husband told me that he awoke in the middle of the night and saw a baby sitting at my feet and reaching for me, laughing and playing. He said, "I thought it was Allie at first, but then Allie was sleeping on the sofa next to you." I felt an excitement swell within me. *Could it be possible? Is this yet another confirmation of our baby's existence?* In some ways, I felt relief because I was not the only one to experience such strange dreams.

Immediately, I recounted my visions to Jack. At first, he seemed to be more impressed with the mysticism of the coincidence than curious about its meaning, but as we discussed it further, we resolved between the two of us that this was God's way of confirming to us the life of our baby. I wouldn't have to spend the rest of my life wondering whether or not I was really pregnant. I could feel at peace with this interpretation, and within my own heart I could accept with serenity that I *really did* have another child. Yet I still refused to emotionally acknowledge my miscarriage.

I wouldn't dare think about her as a miscarriage. Somehow, I just decided that I had a spirit child, not a lost pregnancy. It was easier for me to engage in the impossibility than to face the reality. I didn't have room in my heart to question God or to be angry. It wasn't broken expectations that hurt so much; it was the seeming senselessness of the whole experience. What did it all mean? As Jack said, "What was the point?"

Due to our fears, we never shared our dreams with anyone else. We felt that many of our friends and family would not have understood them or accepted this as a kind of confirmation. Sometimes mysterious things happen, and often we just dismiss them for lack of knowledge about it. The important thing was that Jack and I knew; that's all that seemed to matter.

Three fruitless years passed of us trying to have a baby and being unable to conceive. I started wondering if it would ever happen. We tried fertility drugs, diets, herbal remedies, exercise, and even acupuncture. I was willing to do almost anything to have another child. During those few years, we were both under tremendous amounts of stress.

Jack had found a job at a local video store. Opposite his nighttime hours, I was working mornings at a day care. We were basically spending less than an hour a day with each other. I could see the toll it was taking on our family, especially Allie.

Finally Jack found a new job, one that was in his field of study, graphic design. It called for us to move clear across the country to Minnesota. Though I was glad to leave the memories of Louisiana behind, Jack was leaving all he ever knew. It was a difficult move, but I felt positive about the wonderful changes this new life would bring. I was hopeful that we could finally have another child.

Jack was working late one night, and I heard a voice call, "Momma! Come see!" I ran quickly to the kitchen, thinking my daughter was calling to me at the top of the basement stairs, and I remembered she was in bed asleep. I walked back to her room, and she was indeed sleeping. I felt confused. Did I just imagine that? I clearly heard a voice calling me from the kitchen. Why would I imagine this while I was folding laundry? It didn't make any sense to me. My mind went immediately to the memory of that little girl spirit we would see. I was finally courageous enough to call her my *other* daughter, but only between myself and Jack.

That very night, I decided I was going to write in my journal about what happened three years before. It was time to face my miscarriage for what it really was. I saved the file in my computer under the name Elizabeth. It wasn't something I ever discussed with Jack. I wasn't even entirely sure why I did it.

Why hadn't we ever named her? We never even thought to give her a name; maybe we were afraid to fully accept her. I felt very strongly that I wanted to acknowledge her. I wanted to tell people that I had another daughter. I also felt somewhat guilty, like maybe I seemed ashamed of her; but truly, I wasn't ashamed. I was afraid. I wanted to tell everyone about our little baby girl whom we loved but only ever knew in spirit. But what would people think? I couldn't bear to consider their rejection of her. So I pushed it aside, and for those three years, I tried not to think about her. Finally that night came when I not only acknowledged her, but I had even saved a journal entry under an actual name. When Jack came home, I asked him, "Do you ever think about that spirit we used to see?"

"Yeah, sometimes I still see her. I will think it's Allie, and it turns out she's somewhere else and it couldn't have been."

"Have you ever thought about what her name would be?" In a quick prayer, I thought, *If he says Elizabeth, then that is truly her name.*

"Yeah, a couple of names, I guess." I asked him to tell me the first name that came to his mind. "Elizabeth."

I gasped for air several times, as if someone was trying to take the air from me. How? How could he say that? We never talked about it. We never even mentioned other names for girls. I asked him to get my computer and open the document folder. There he saw a file named Elizabeth.

His first reaction was not very different from the night we discussed our dreams. His eyes widened, and he seemed impressed with the coincidence. I told him to open it, and there he found all that I had typed about my memories of our first miscarriage. He said, "Well, that must be her name." He seemed so calm, as if these inexplicable events were common. I was the one that was astounded, out of my own breath. After her name was given to us, I felt even more relief. Now we could say her name to one another, and secretly, we could always call her that.

In November of 2007, I received a message from someone I went to high school with. I only knew her vaguely, but she remembered me, and we started e-mailing and talking on the phone. She had lost a pregnancy as well, and I finally felt safe enough to tell someone about our Elizabeth. I knew she would understand, and as she listened, I began to realize that acknowledging my daughter brought to me a new healing in my spirit. It helped me so much just to say her name aloud to someone else. I was surprised to find out that many of my feelings of guilt and denial were very normal and that other women also felt the way I did. They also felt isolated and hushed by the world about something that was so deeply a part of them. From that moment on, I wanted to make a way for women to share their story and to have something to hold on to, to say, "This child was a part of me and is now a part of heaven," and as soon as I became willing, God made the way.

I arrived to exercise one morning and found a flyer at the YMCA about a Christian miscarriage support group. I called them, not really knowing what I wanted to say, but after our first meeting, I felt alive again. The women truly understood my feelings. They had even experienced visions themselves, regarding their lost babies. I was ecstatic!

The realization that I was not alone in my feelings, in my fears, or even in my baby-related dreams was more than I needed to give me peace. I felt so empowered by this peace coming from the acknowledgement of my secret baby, Elizabeth, that I decided to go through my first miscarriage Bible study. I had a purpose and a drive inside me. I felt God light me up on the inside, and I was sure that Elizabeth could be an inspiration, not a secret and hidden shame anymore. This freedom inspired me.

CHAPTER THREE

At the time I began the first of my three miscarriage-related Bible studies, there were no other women in the group, except for the director and myself. Doing a one-on-one study with a perfect stranger about a very personal secret was way beyond my comfort zone. It had to be God that empowered me to walk through those doors.

I felt very nervous entering class that day with my workbook in hand. I really didn't feel the need to take the class, except with the hopes of teaching it. I felt certain that I had dealt with all my miscarriage pain, when really all I had done was found a way to live around it. The director, Ronda, and I got along great. During the first meeting, we practically lost track of time becoming instant friends. I was ready to prove to her and to myself that I could easily go through this Bible study.

Throughout the next week, I looked through the study, realizing it was much more difficult to answer the questions than I expected. Pretty soon the entire week had gone by, and I had barely finished the first chapter; this happened nearly every week. The night before each class, I would rush to fill in the blanks. At class the next day, I would review my answers with Ronda. Yet the amazing part about my first Bible study was when we sat discussing each question and verse, I felt the peace of God enter the room. I could sense his presence, almost as if we were sitting at his feet having a talk with him. This feeling repeated itself at every class, in every study, but somehow I still found it difficult during the week to face the questions in the book.

Many of the questions were designed to get the reader to confront their grief. I kept telling Ronda that I didn't think it applied to my miscarriage but that I could relate to it in other ways. For nearly five weeks, it was the same thing at each class. I'd answer the questions, avoiding the miscarriage as much as possible, applying the grief questions to the loss of my parents. Yet there was an unrecognizable heaviness that seemed to be slowly easing by each passing week. There was a part of me that needed healing that I didn't even know existed.

Midway through the study, I had an epiphany. Elizabeth's purpose! I knew the answer to Jack's question, "What was the point?" I had found it. I felt sure the reason I miscarried was so I could come to this moment, working through this specific study to find God in my life in a completely new way. I was also meant to find healing from the unresolved grief of losing my parents.

I thought to myself about all those methods I used as I tried to get through the loss of my parents. I had tried counseling, moving from place to place, changing churches, changing friendships, changing myself. I never got over the feelings of abandonment that their losses left in my life. I never accepted their departure. I tried to replace their loss with the empty fulfillment of others in my life. I was caught in an endless circle of seeking and being disappointed.

This was just like my infertility and my miscarriage! The feelings of abandonment, loss, fear, and even replacement. Oh, how we tried to have another child after losing Elizabeth. What had started out as hope for another addition had become an obsession, one that I didn't even realize was taking over my mind and my family as well. Nothing seemed good enough. Nothing filled that empty need.

As I finished up the study, I began to wonder if I had only uncovered *part* of the reason God had taken our Elizabeth back to heaven. I felt good knowing that her spirit existed to help me find healing, but I also felt a sense of unfinished business with the study. I knew there had to be more purpose for her existence than just that, and I questioned God about it. In his mysterious way, he led me to the following two verses.

> Just as you cannot understand the path of the wind or the mystery of a tiny baby growing in its mother's womb, so you cannot understand the activity of God, who does all things.
>
> Ecclesiastes 11:5

> "My thoughts are nothing like your thoughts," says the Lord. "And my ways are far beyond anything you could imagine. For just as the heavens are higher than the earth, so my ways are higher than your ways and my thoughts higher than your thoughts."
>
> Isaiah 55:8–9

I realized that fully understanding God's choices is not always an option, but I still continued to search for an answer because until I was satisfied I would not find peace.

By following the Bible study, I was able to gain an incredible understanding of Elizabeth's spirit, which in and of itself was very healing to me. When I read Jeremiah 1:5, "I knew you before I formed you in your mother's womb. Before you were born I set you apart and appointed you as my prophet to the nations," I felt God speaking to me. I also heard his voice when I read in Psalms:

> You made all the delicate, inner parts of my body and knit me together in my mother's womb. Thank you for making me so wonderfully complex! Your workmanship is marvelous—how well I know it. You watched me as I was being formed in utter seclusion, as I was woven together in the dark of the womb. You saw me before I was born. Every day of my life was recorded in your book. Every moment was laid out before a single day had passed.
>
> Psalm 139:13–16

By reading these verses, I could at least begin to understand the way our Elizabeth's spirit entered into existence. I could see that God knew Elizabeth before she even existed in my womb. God allowed me to be the "nostrils" (so to speak) that he used to breathe life into her being. He used my body as a portal to create her exact spirit for his exact purpose, and though her spirit was not meant for a body, it was meant for something greater on the other side of heaven. I can now see what a blessing and a privilege it has been to be the means by which God chose to bring this extraordinary spirit into existence and almost immediately into heaven.

Despite the fact that I constantly tried to make the Bible study about the loss of my parents, God kept revealing truths to me anyway. One of the most important truths that I discovered in regard to my parents' loss, as well as the loss of Elizabeth, was that they did not stop existing the day they left this earth. They did not stay stuck in the same time and place when and where it happened; they're not floating around, lost in space. I was the one stuck. I was the one floating around, lost in time and space.

Sometimes I wondered if I had left my loved ones behind, but I was the one being left as they moved on to what their purpose was and is. They kept existing; they kept living; why should I stop? If anything, they have begun to live in ways that I have yet to experience! They're not only okay where they are, they are amazing, fulfilling their God-given destiny. Just because I can't wrap my mind around God's exact purpose and reason doesn't mean that a purpose doesn't exist.

CHAPTER FOUR

Equipped with the knowledge and power of the first Bible study, I was confident that life was headed in a new direction. I committed to embark on co-facilitating the next support group meeting so I could learn how to effectively teach the class, but before we even began, I was celebrating a new miracle. After four years of infertility, I was finally pregnant again. I was so proud of my new blessing that I told everyone I met about our little one on the way. I was in shock for the first week, feeling as if I were living on the outside of a dream. Although this dream-state never seemed to end, the utter bliss did begin to fade when I suddenly realized that I was on a timeline. I had to live through eight more uncertain weeks in order to know my baby would make it. Those eight weeks were the most horrible of my adult life. What started as a little concern slowly turned into absolute terror. Jack seemed to be in state of shock. He was happy and pleased with the surprise, but after four years of trying to get pregnant, the unexpected news flabbergasted both of us.

I felt so overwhelmed by my fear of losing this

baby that I began to disconnect with her and with God. Something seemed off, but I tried to ignore those feelings. I became consumed with fear and anxiety.

Meanwhile, the second miscarriage-related Bible study began. Though I felt as if I didn't have very much to offer to the class, I still attended. It seemed as if my lessons from the first class had gone out the window, and I was functioning more on a kind of autopilot. I felt humbled and embarrassed at my obvious weakness in spirit; I was so easily moved from that remarkable closeness to God.

I still couldn't believe I was pregnant. I hated that I had to remind myself. I lived in a constant state of fear. Four years I dreamed of what it would be like to be pregnant again, yet I kept thinking, *This isn't how it's supposed to be.* It felt so unreal. There were times during those beginning weeks that I sometimes wished I wasn't pregnant. How? How could I think such things? I hated myself for thinking it, but the anxiety and fear began to actually hurt. For so long, being pregnant was my sincerest desire. We wanted another baby. I was sure this was meant to be, but something about it didn't seem right.

Jack could sense my tension, and we were most definitely very edgy with one another. We stopped and questioned ourselves, "Why are we fighting? What is happening to our family?" Well, I did eventually make it to my twelve-week mark, and I felt an amazing sense of relief. *Oh thank goodness, we're safe*, I thought. *I have to stop all this worrying.* The tension eased up a bit, and I started connecting with our baby.

When I first found out I was pregnant, I bought a journal to keep for this baby. I had made a pregnancy journal for Allie and have plans to give it to her when she is older. It only seemed fair to keep a pregnancy journal for this child as well.

(Four weeks, six days)
Hello, little baby. So we just found out yesterday about you! Here's my first reaction, screaming, "What? What?" Then the trembling. "Oh my God! Thank you, God!" Let me tell you how very ecstatic we are about your arrival. We have prayed for you, waited for you, and wanted you in our family for so long. Four years ago, your big sister Elizabeth went to heaven, only a few weeks older than you are now. And we have awaited your arrival ever since! However, I'm just not very patient, my little one. I was rushing God. I was going to fertility specialists and taking medicine, but you never came. Finally I let go of all my pressure, and I realized that God wanted me to rely on him and his timing, not just on what I wanted. So I let go, and now you are on your way! Well, you're here inside me, you are growing and changing, and I feel so amazing and scared and thrilled all at the same time. I love you so much already. Well, of course, as your mother, that's not hard to believe. I will love you always now. I am your mother now and forever. I am so ready to hold you! But you just keep on growing strong, my sweet one. We'll touch when it's time!

Your big sister Alicen is very shocked and confused about you. She doesn't know what to expect. But today, she was giggling about you. After our dog Kodee stepped on my stomach, Allie laughed and said, "She's just saying hello to the baby."

Daddy is in full take-care-of-things mode. Taking care of me and finishing old projects, what a little motivator you already are! May-May and Poppy could just about burst with excitement. People are already wondering what you are, boy or girl. We love you no matter what!

Kisses and lovin, Momma

(Five weeks, two days)
Hello! We had an ultrasound today. They want me to come back a week from tomorrow, since your heartbeat didn't show. I was a little disappointed, but they said you're just too early to show that. I love you. I will have to wait patiently though, so I will, and hopefully we'll see your little heart beating away next time. How can I describe how tired I am? I know, like the feeling right before you doze off, only all the time. I'm too tired to focus.

Love and kisses, Momma

P.S. Your sister nicknamed you Sammi. We have no idea where she gets it, but maybe time will tell. We love you, Sammi!

It is so difficult for me to read through these journal entries. It tears me up inside just thinking about those days.

Between weeks seven and eight, I had a major problem. I went to the bathroom, to discover what seemed to be the start of a period. I feared the worst. I was certain I was beginning to miscarry. I yelled for Jack, and he rushed me to the ER. The ride over was a time full of prayer. We were pleading with God for this baby, asking for acceptance of his will but also for his mercy and grace to allow our child to come healthy and happy into our arms.

When we arrived to the doctors, they did an ultrasound and decided that I had two placental hemorrhages. They told me that it would heal on its own, and we went home praying they were right. The one benefit of this unexpected trip to the hospital was that we were finally able to see the baby's heart beating perfectly.

By week ten I was very sick. I had the stomach flu, and I could not get my energy up. Everyone kept telling me that it was completely normal to be so drained, but I kept questioning why it was so severe. I told Jack that after this baby was born I never wanted to be pregnant again. I couldn't take being so sick so much of the time.

I still felt scared and nervous about losing the baby. I didn't want to worry, and I felt like God was helping me face my fears, but emotionally and spiritually, I was tired and in need of a refreshing recharge. Twelve weeks finally arrived, and I felt some comfort, but underlying worries still filled my heart. I kept praying and begging God to let my baby be all right.

The Bible study lasted nine weeks, and by the end of the study, it was time for a memorial service. I had not done a memorial for Elizabeth and kept putting it off. Ronda hoped I would do Elizabeth's memorial with the other mother going through the study, but I couldn't. For the other mom's memorial service, we went to her son's grave. He was stillborn at nearly full term. I stood to the right of his grave, with my head bowed, unable to speak or even look them in the eye. I could feel their sorrow, but I didn't want to understand it. I was relieved when the second Bible study ended. It was too much worry for me. I could not tolerate the reminders that my own pregnancy might not end successfully.

At that point, I began pulling away from God. Inside I could feel a budding resentment toward him. I knew that he could take my baby from me at any time, and I struggled within myself as I found it more and more difficult to face God. It seemed there had been a wall built between us, but I didn't want to lose the closeness I had found during the first study.

It wasn't only God that I was blaming. I was ashamed, and I blamed myself. I kept wondering, *How could I have saved my Elizabeth? How can I save this baby? I don't listen to the signals. I should know when something isn't right. Maybe I did feel it with Elizabeth, and I didn't do anything about it.*

In that moment, God seemed to urge me to reevaluate my views of life and death. He reminded me of a verse, "I am the one who kills and gives life; I am the one who wounds and heals" (Deuteronomy 32:39b). I needed to be thinking about who does the creating of life and where he begins knowing us and loving us. He also reminded me that he knew her before he even formed her in my womb, by pointing me to Jeremiah 1:5.

As I faced the truth that I did not physically cause her death, I began to question whether or not I was being punished. I asked God what I had done to cause him to take his blessing away from me. In that moment

I was given a reminder of the poor blind man in the gospel of John. Jesus said, "It was not because of his sins or his parents' sins, This happened so the power of God could be seen in him" (John 9:3).

I decided that I would sit down and write God a letter. While writing, I received a vision in my mind of a wall. I was asking God about it, asking for how I could get over the wall. I never considered the possibility of the answer. I saw Jesus lifting the wall and taking it away. I never even thought the wall could be removed. Here is my letter as I wrote it to God, at thirteen weeks along.

> Lord, I know that I have been distant from you and this baby for some time. I partly feel this is due to fear and certainly a great deal of spiritual warfare. When I was feeling so down, one thing seemed to pile on top of another, and I didn't have the energy to get up under it all. But Lord, I sincerely miss our meetings, all those special talks that you and I would have, when I knew I would be in your holy presence. It was a sense of peace and love and a cozy warmth that seemed to radiate into my words as I prayed back to you in response. I also miss that sense of closeness with you. Knowing I can call at any time, and maybe it's a lie to myself to feel so hindered in calling on you now, but I do feel strongly that there is a wall between us. Lord, I can speculate all day as to why I feel so far from you, but the truth is that it comes down to me, and the one thing I need to do is to quit avoiding you.

I'm scared to say, "I'm ready to face the wall," because I don't truly want to. Lord, I am still at least going to try. I know that my desire to sit right next to you is stronger than my fear of the hurt and tears that wall may bring. So I'm coming to you, asking you to take the burden of the wall away. If I can give you my fears of losing this baby the way I lost Elizabeth, then I know I will find a better healing.

I know, God, that this baby, Sammi, is yours. You take this burden of fear and help me let go of control. I am offering up to you again the unseen child that I so desperately love already. If you have this baby return to you, then I know it is safely in your arms. Lord, my mind might not be in it, but you can know in my heart I hear your call and I acknowledge that it must be done. I know Abraham waited many years more than four to have his child, and I know it must have been hard for him to offer that child, Isaac, back to you, but if it isn't now, we will have to offer them to you sometime. I would rather Sammi be safely in your hands in heaven than to have my baby here with me, against your will.

Lord, I put Alicen, Elizabeth, and Sammi in your hands. I give you my children. I trust that your ability to guide them is far superior to mine, and I pray, no I beg you, to keep them always in your pathways. I ask that their lives be fulfilled in the end by joining you in heaven, eternally, as Elizabeth already has. I pray that you heal my heart and fill the holes left by her lack of physical presence in my life. I pray that you release me from the grip of darkness that takes advantage of my weakness and vulnerability when it comes to my children. I pray in Jesus' name.

Though I felt more connected to God after coming to him so sincerely in prayer, I still felt there was something amiss with this pregnancy. I could not figure out what it was, so I tried to ignore it. I kept telling myself that I was paranoid.

Week fourteen of my pregnancy was really something special. It was the first time I felt Sammi flutter inside me. We also began feeling a hard ball shape in my lower abdomen. The shape seemed to move, and we assumed it was the baby moving. We were excited to be able to start connecting with the baby. It gave us so much hope, and it seemed to be a sign to stop worrying.

I also began to notice an excited tickle feeling when Allie would come barreling her face into my stomach, saying, "Good night, Sammi!" The feeling seemed to come also when Jack played his guitar. We felt all these things were ways of connecting with Sammi. We thought maybe we needed to forget the worries and start living as if this baby would really arrive. So we decided to start getting ready for Sammi.

Allie was going to have to share her room, so we ordered her a new bed. She was thrilled. She told everyone at school that the baby would be in her room. Jack bought me a new baby bag for my birthday, and Allie had chosen the baby a first-year scrapbook.

At seventeen weeks, though, I was feeling pretty

lousy physically. I was concerned that the feelings of tiredness were not going away, and something seemed to really be wrong. I had some spotting and decided to go in to be checked.

CHAPTER FIVE

At my seventeen-week appointment, I felt a sense of longing for an ultrasound. I tried to ignore the feeling because I was afraid the staff would think I was just trying to rush my eighteen-week ultrasound. Even though I had started spotting again, which had been happening on and off all throughout the pregnancy, they didn't seem too concerned. As the nurse held the digital heartbeat monitor to my stomach, all we could hear was static and occasionally my own heartbeat. She said, "I am registering the baby's heartbeat. See?" Then she pointed the monitor toward me.

Personally, I didn't see any numbers, but I wanted to believe her, "Well, if you see it registering..."

"Well, the baby is moving so much I can't get a heartbeat on the speaker, but it is registering. Wait, there it is. No, now it's gone." She moved the monitor around. "Here, here it is. Did you hear it? The baby must have moved again." I laughed and thought, *Well, if she's moving this much, then she's okay.* Something told me to ask for an ultrasound then, but I knew they would deny my request.

However, a few days later, I developed a sick feeling in my heart. I told Jack, "I don't think this baby is going to make it to the end of my pregnancy, and I'm not sure if I will either." I hated to confess my fears aloud. Secretly, I thought if I admitted them then I was somehow going to curse myself, and then it would be my fault if something happened. Jack tried to reassure me that everything was okay, but I couldn't be convinced.

By the time I was eighteen and a half weeks, I really had a hard time convincing myself everything was okay. Jack wasn't the only one trying to convince me; the doctors, our friends, and family all told me I was fine, despite my feelings of uneasiness. But they were all wrong. September 4, 2008, after Allie went to bed, I was taking a soak in the tub. When I stood up, I felt a rush of hot liquid come out of me. My water broke, though at the time I wasn't sure what had happened. I called our insurance nurse hotline, and they suggested I call the doctor immediately.

I called the doctor, almost apologetically, embarrassed to be the annoying client that calls constantly after hours. The doctor scared me when she said, "Oh. Oh…I hope this isn't what I think it is. You need to have an ultrasound right now."

I called a friend to come and sit with Allie so she wouldn't have to wake up and come with us to the emergency room. When I arrived and explained what happened, they didn't seem too worried. The nurse was sure that she could just get out the monitor, find the heartbeat, prove to me that I was just a worrywart, and then I would go home, embarrassed at my senseless concern. Maybe this is what I was hoping for as well.

The nurse couldn't find the heartbeat, but I wasn't concerned about that too much because the week before the other nurse couldn't get it on the speaker but was able to register it through the digital monitor. The nurse then said, "I don't use these very often; let me get someone else to try." I could hear her talking to the doctor in the hallway, and then she went into a whisper. Sickened by this turn of events, I knew what it all meant, but I wouldn't accept it. The doctor tried for the heartbeat. His eyes were kind and pitiful, but I was getting angry.

"I'm sorry, Kristie. I can't find the heartbeat." The proud nurse's face melted to humble pity. She grabbed my hand and rubbed my arm as the doctor kept trying for a heartbeat.

"No," I said. "No, your monitor isn't working. The nurse last week couldn't get it on the speaker either, but she said it registered in her monitor. Your monitor isn't digital. You need another one. That isn't the kind I need."

"Kristie, there's nothing wrong with it. This monitor works. I'm afraid—"

"You're wrong. I want an ultrasound." I started to cry.

"You definitely need one, but we don't have that available right now. You will have to come back in the morning to get an ultrasound."

I burst into angry tears. I felt utter hatred for this wretched hospital and their inadequacy. I had no choice except to leave. I went home, and my friend asked how it went. Bursting into tears again, I blurted out, "They think the baby died!" (Notice I said *they* think.) I was furious with them for not offering me hope.

My friend clearly didn't know what to say. What

could be said? She sighed. "Oh no. I'm sorry." She left and went home wishing me well for the morning ultrasound.

Jack came in and said we needed to try and get some sleep. We didn't speak much that night. I lay in the bed for as long as I could keep my eyes open. I don't remember falling asleep, but I was ready first thing in the morning to go and prove the doctor wrong. I just kept hoping that the baby was still alive and they would be able to explain this all to me.

The next morning, I went in for an ultrasound at 9:00 a.m. When I arrived for the appointment, nervously, I jokingly said, "Well, at least we get to see how much the baby has grown. Last time, she was only the size of a grain of rice."

The technician said soberly, "You can't watch the ultrasound, and I can't tell you anything."

I was upset by this shocking approach to my ultrasound. "Well, can't you tell me if the baby's heart is beating?"

"No."

"Can't you tell me if the baby is even moving?"

"No, I can't tell you anything."

"Well fine! Jack, watch the screen close!"

She took her measurements and quickly left the room. Jack stood at my feet, and his eyes watered as he mouthed to me, "The baby's not moving."

I was angry that he was ready to give up. "Well, *you* don't know how to read an ultrasound!" Another technician returned to take one photo, and I just knew it was of the baby's heart. I knew this wasn't a good sign. In my mind, however, I told myself, *Maybe the baby has a problem with her heart. We can deal with anything, just not death.* I prayed that she would be healed from her sickness. They gave me a CD of the ultrasound to take to my doctor, who was an hour's drive away.

When I arrived at the clinic, there was a mix-up on what time I would be arriving, and I had to wait until twelve thirty to meet with the doctor. I kept seeing nurses grab my red folder, open it, and put it back on the shelf. It was as if no one wanted to be the one to take me to the back.

When the doctor finally walked in, she said, "I'm so sorry about the results."

"What results?" My eyes widened; my heart pounded hard and quick in my throat.

"Oh! They didn't tell you?" I shook my head no. "The baby died."

Just like that. It was so definite. My gut heaved as I gasped for air. In my tears, I felt nothing but complete destruction. She went on talking. "I'm so sorry. Now, we'll need to send you over to have you induced. Well, we could do surgery if you wanted, but then the baby would have to come out in pieces…" She went on and on explaining the process ahead of me, but I was still stuck at her first statement, "The baby died."

"No," I interrupted, "the equipment there, it's not reliable. We have to check again."

Sympathetically, she scheduled me for an ultrasound at their hospital. This time the technician confirmed to us, "No, I'm sorry, there is no heartbeat." I just cried. The doctor explained to me that I would be given my own personal nurse when I went in to deliver, so they scheduled me to come back later that night to be admitted. I went home for a few hours, wondering all the way home how I would tell my five-year-old daughter that our Sammi was gone.

She was so excited about the baby coming. She was

completely ready to be a big sister. I remember how she'd come over and jiggle my belly just to hear me say, "Stop! You're making Sammi dizzy!" Then she would laugh hysterically. She was even the one to name the baby. I remember her telling my stomach, "Goodnight, Sammi!" I thought about how during the day she would nuzzle my stomach and say, "I love you, Sammi!" All of those joy-filled memories were nothing but heartache now. We would never have our Sammi to live to tell these to. Sammi would never be old enough to hear the giggly bedtime stories of how much her big sister loved her, even when she was in my tummy.

We arrived at the sitter's house to pick Allie up. I couldn't look my friend in the eye. I felt ashamed of myself, humiliated at my own inability to carry a baby. When we came home, we told Allie that we had some very sad news. "Sammi's soul has gone to heaven, and Mommy has to go to the hospital tonight. Daddy will be at home with you, and Mommy will be back home soon." She looked baffled.

"Is Sammi in your tummy?"

"No, my baby, Sammi is in heaven now."

But she didn't understand. All she kept saying was, "But why, Momma?" The last words she said to me before I left for the hospital were, "Momma, why did our baby's soul have to go to heaven?" I was heartbroken. What answer would be enough? None.

My mentor, Mrs. Gayle, met us at home when we returned from the clinic that afternoon and helped us get things together as we mentally tried to prepare for the delivery. She took Allie for a walk to the park while we packed my bags. Then Ronda, arrived to pick me up and bring me to the hospital. She was going to stay with me for a while there. One of Jack's closest family friends, Stacie, was on her way from her home, three hours away, to also be at the hospital with me.

Jack and I both agreed that one of us needed to be with Allie and that the best thing for her was to stay home and to stay in her routine. She had never slept away from home, and we didn't want this time to be her first experience with it. If she were to become scared or upset, we would be too far away to comfort her. So Jack stayed home with Allie, and I went to the hospital with these two women who sincerely understood what I was going through.

We parked by the emergency room, which was very crowded that night. The man at the front desk was not concerned with my heartache or my privacy. I asked for the nurse, as instructed, and he blurted out (very loudly I might add), "Well, are you pregnant? How far along are you?"

I replied quietly, "I'm eighteen and a half weeks. I was told to ask for the nurse to come get me from labor and delivery. I'm miscarrying."

His response was cold as he turned to an ER nurse who stood by the desk, getting papers. "Can you help her? She's eighteen weeks and miscarrying. She says she wants to go to labor and delivery!"

He said it incredibly loud, and I was humiliated. Didn't I have a patient's right to privacy? I felt like all eyes were on me. I turned my sorrows inward, not making eye contact with anyone.

The nurse's response was not much better than his. "No! She needs to fill out that pink form; you can't go upstairs." She looked at me, disgusted.

By this point, I was nearly irate. "Yes, I can!" My speech sped up. "I was told to come to the desk. There would be a note. You're supposed to call the nurse so that I can go upstairs!"

The nurse finally realized the doctor had already arranged all of this and said without any sense of feeling, "Oh, you need to go to the front desk." And she walked away.

"I don't know where that is from here—"

Before I could finish my sentence, the man interrupted me, saying, "Well, I'm going to *tell* you how!" He gave me directions, looked at me stupidly, as if I couldn't understand his words, and mortified, I walked away.

At this bewildering point, I began putting up walls. My humiliation seemed to crush me. *It's the beginning of Sammi's rejection, just like Elizabeth. I knew it.* The sense that other people didn't care about my losing a child due to miscarriage was for me the hardest part about grieving. It wasn't as if they didn't completely care; it was just *how* they belittled my grief. It was the idea that miscarriage isn't as bad as losing a real person. Their lack of recognition of my deep sorrow created a feeling of insecurity in me as I grieved. I thought, *Here we go again with people not understanding or giving value to my child's life.*

My baby meant nothing to that man at the desk or the nurse behind him. It was a cruel, harsh feeling. Just as it should be anytime someone doesn't value a human life. I don't understand how they could treat my child's life so lightly, as if it didn't matter that my baby died. It's barbaric. I tried to tell others that just a week and a half longer and she would have been considered stillborn. I thought, *Then they might give value to my loss.* But it didn't matter. No one seemed to understand, except the other women who had experienced this sorrow.

When we arrived at the other front desk, I immediately noticed the yellow note, and the difference was amazing. They were so kind and compassionate, obviously waiting for me. Ronda told them about my horrible first encounter. I probably wouldn't have mentioned it, just because I was so traumatized by the entirety of what I was about to go through. The receptionist apologized profusely, but it didn't erase my experience by any means. Later, several nurses, including the head of the labor and delivery department, came by to offer apologies.

My first nurse came down to meet with us; she took us up a private elevator, which was intended to avoid passing in front of the nursery. I was admitted to the labor and delivery floor. I went up to my room at 7:30 p.m. By 9:15 p.m., I was given my first dose of medicine to soften my cervix. As Stacie arrived, I introduced her to Ronda. They were instantly friends. The nurses actually thought we were all related for how close we were during this terrible time. No one else can ever know what those few hours meant or what we shared with one another during that time. No one would ever know what kind of bond that experience would create in my heart for these women, one that will last for the rest of my life.

I was surprised that I was not feeling the effects of the medicine, but by 1:15 a.m., I was starting to cramp a bit. They gave me my next dose, and we all decided to try to get some sleep. At 5:00 a.m., I was awakened by intense cramping. It seemed to come in waves. I hesitated to call the nurse because I didn't want to wake everyone else up, but I couldn't stand the pain anymore.

When she came in to check on me, I told her the cramping was really bad. She asked if I wanted ibuprofen, and I said I didn't know. She talked to the doctor, and the doctor explained that I need not endure *any* pain during this and they were to give me anything I wanted to ease it. She asked if I was ready for my epidural. I thought I would try to wait a while, but by 5:45 a.m., I was unable to tolerate it any longer. She had the anesthesiologist come in at 6:00 a.m. for my epidural. They kept telling me, "He's really fast; he's known for that." I thought, *Good.* However, I soon found out that speed versus quality is definitely not worth it.

He came in and gave me a shot in my back to numb the area, but he did not wait for the shot to take effect before he jammed the tube into my spine. I will never forget that resistant feeling as he shoved the tube into my back; I screamed and trembled in pain. Imagine the feeling of someone pushing a straw through Styrofoam. This would be the equivalent to how it felt as he shoved the tube into my spine. My blood pressure was fluctuating, and I was shaking uncontrollably from the intense pain and horror of what just happened. They kept asking, "Are you cold?" I was in more pain than I was cold, but in a way, deep down inside, my spirit did feel cold. I felt a part of me die that night.

By 6:20 a.m., I was feeling things coming out of me. I was on my left side facing Stacie, and Ronda was at my feet. The nurse said that it was everything beginning to pass through and that I would feel that sensation for a while. I said, "It's coming! I have to turn over. My baby will *not* be born on my side." The nurse didn't think it was happening that fast. Yet, at 6:23 a.m., when I turned over, I felt my baby roll out of me.

My emotions erupted like an enormous dam bursting open, echoing my massive heartache as my baby lay dead on my bed. Stacie leapt toward me and wrapped me in her arms as I cried and wailed, turning back to my left side. I refused to look until they had cleaned my baby. I didn't want to see her covered in blood. Initially, they told me they would dress her so I could spend time with her. The doctors came in, and Stacie assured me I could turn over and that I wouldn't see anything until I was ready. I remember asking, "What is it? Is it a boy or a girl?"

The doctor turned to me and said, "We can't tell. It could be either way. The baby has shrunk a little due to lack of blood flow and is too small to tell. Possibly a girl. We won't be able to dress the baby; it's too small." I felt numb from that very moment. Someone had pulled a plug inside me. All emotion drained from my face, and I felt nothing. It seemed cruel. Why wouldn't my Sammi be big enough for the dignity of being dressed? I couldn't imagine what I would see when they handed me my child. Was she deformed? Was she human looking?

CHAPTER SIX

I held on to Stacie for dear life. She asked me if I wanted her to see what Sammi looked like so she could prepare me. They told me what I would see and warned me that Sammi's color was different. They explained how Sammi's head had become compressed from resting down in me so low for so long without life. They estimated that she died at about sixteen weeks. They covered Sammi's head as they laid my baby's body onto my lap.

Initially, all I wanted was to see my baby's hands and feet, but when I saw those tiny fingers and toes and I saw those skinny little legs and arms, I lifted the blanket. I had to see my Sammi's face. Her head was not perfectly round in the back, due to the compression, but her face was perfect. I stared at her teeny little nose and mouth, her tiny eyes, jawline, and chin. She was so small. I wondered, *How could something be so perfect and so gone?* How could we have come so far and lose her then? Everyone stood away from me, on the other side of the delivery room, giving me the time I needed as I held her fragile body. I was afraid to touch her skin because it was so thin and transparent. "Okay, that's enough," I said.

They put her in the warmer, and I called Jack. Then I asked them to take her body away. I agreed to have testing done so I could prevent this tragedy from happening again, hoping to gain some clue as to why this happened. They warned me that even with the testing most people never know what happened.

I never will forget what my child looked like. Some people would rather think of miscarriage as a glob of tissue. They would rather not face that idea that a life of an innocent human being is gone. They would have to ask God why, and that's often too unbearable to think about. But I saw her. She was real, she was human, she was mine, and I wanted her to live.

I was just as saddened to lose Elizabeth as I was Sammi. It's funny how many people ask you to compare your depth of sorrow for an eighteen-and-a-half week loss to an eight-week loss. Yes, I had to face delivery and a funeral for Sammi, but did my love and grief vary with the loss of one child over another? Of course not! I saw both my children. I held my Sammi, and even though we only saw my Elizabeth fleetingly, do I sorrow less? Do I remember their bodies any less? Different as they were, they were still each a child of mine.

Ronda left that morning close to 8:00 a.m., and I assured her I was fine. Jack arrived around 9:30 a.m., and Stacie stayed another half hour. Before Jack arrived, I was sitting up in bed, trying my best to get up and go to the bathroom. The epidural had made my legs quite useless. I asked Stacie, "Please help me. I really have to go." She put her arms under mine and helped me take two steps from the bed, but I nearly passed out.

She called the nurse for me, and I said, "If you don't help me get there, then you will have a bigger problem right here." They brought in a bedside toilet. We struggled to get me over, and before I knew it, the emotional strain of what had just happened to me hit my system and it emptied itself of everything in one swift blow. It was so intense that I completely passed out.

As I came back to some awareness, the nurses were saying, "Kristie, look at me. Kristie, open your eyes." I grunted in acknowledgement, hoping that would be good enough.

When I finally came back to full consciousness, I remember saying over and over, "I'm okay. I feel better. I'm okay." The nurses giggled at me. I don't even know why I was saying it, but over and over, I kept saying, "I feel better. I'm okay." Inside, I did feel an urgency, a need to be okay, and I also felt strangely numb. I know I talked to people that day, and I know that more things happened, but it just seemed to be nothing. It all felt like nothing at that point.

Later that same day, the nurses that had bonded so well with us each said their good-byes, and one left with a promise to pray for me. The final nurse came in, gave me a tearful good-bye, and presented me with a multitude of tiny blessings. She cried as she said, "I'm just so sad about what you are going to have to go through." She gave me a baby-sized bracelet that one of the nurses made with the letters of Sammi's name in beads. Also, she gave me a certificate of life with Sammi's feet and handprints. These are things I will treasure all the rest of my life.

After I seemed to be feeling a little better, I was wheeled down to the front entrance where Jack picked me up, and we went home. The first thing I saw as I walked into the bedroom was the rocking chair. I lost it. "Get that out of here! I can't be in here with that! I don't want that chair in this room! Get it out! I can't have this room looking like this. I can't take it looking the same as when Sammi was inside me. I won't sleep in here until it looks different." I hurried back to the sofa and cried. Jack quickly moved the chair, and I crawled into bed, crying.

Later that evening, I looked in the fridge and saw some food I had cooked two days before. I wanted to throw up when I realized I was still pregnant when I cooked it. I didn't want to see anything that reminded me of being pregnant or any reminders to me of how happy we felt to have a baby with us. I told Jack that I wanted to put all of her things in the casket and bury them with her: her journal, her bibs, that book Allie bought, even the diaper bag he gave me for my birthday. I just couldn't face it. Nevertheless, I'm glad we did not get rid of her things. I am glad we didn't erase her from our lives. At the time, I wanted my memories to be fast-forwarded, but everything seemed a reminder of when I was pregnant.

I remember Jack kneeling by the bed as I cried, stroking my forehead softly. "Baby, you're going to have to face these things. You're going to have to eventually face all of these firsts. You can't put it off." Everything was a first. A first bath not being pregnant, a first meal at home not being pregnant. A first time seeing someone since I was pregnant, a first time smiling, a first time laughing—nothing would ever be the same, and I felt lost in that tornado of firsts, leaving a path of complete confusion in its wake. When you make changes in life, you can slowly ease into those changes with time to process and think about all the aspects. But I was forced suddenly, cold-turkey, into being a recently pregnant mother now without a baby.

The next day, I felt like I needed our pets to be home with us, so we drove to pick them up from the pet-sitter. I didn't feel sick physically, and I didn't feel sore, only a little crampy but nothing severe. Mentally, I felt as if I had been warped back in time and twisted all around. I was not pregnant anymore. Life was not about Sammi's arrival anymore, but I felt some contentment to hold our three-month-old kitten. He fit right into that empty place in my arms. One night, I was holding him as he purred himself to sleep on my stomach. I stood up, carrying him to my room, and suddenly I realized that this was a kitten and it was not my baby. My empty arms wanted my baby, not a cat! That's when I knew the depth of my pain.

Immediately, I started planning Sammi's funeral. I started to busy myself with things, and people kept looking at me wondering, "Why are you doing this? You need to rest and give yourself time." What they didn't understand is that time doesn't make it better. Time is painful and slow when someone dies. I hated time. I despised it for being the only cure to my pain.

The details fell into place; the date for the funeral was set, and Sammi's casket was chosen. I made a small silk quilt to lay over her casket, purple and white to match the teddy bear they gave me at the hospital. We made bookmarks and had them printed and laminated. When I first arrived to the hospital, they gave me a teddy bear, which we now call "Sammi bear." Allie drew a picture of the teddy bear, and we made this a part of the bookmark for her funeral.

At home, Allie seemed to be doing okay. But when she would start being naughty, I would correct her, and then she would go into a fit of rage. She would scream and cry that she didn't like me anymore. I told her how hurtful that was, and I asked her what was making her so angry. She told me that I was "mean for going to the hospital and leaving Sammi there." In her mind, I abandoned Sammi. The idea torments me.

"I love our baby," I assured her. "I would never leave Sammi, but she died. I didn't want her to die. I wanted her to live and to come home to us. I wanted the same thing you wanted, but I couldn't stop death. I couldn't make it better." I was humbled to admit that Mommy didn't have all the answers and scared to let her know that some things even mommies and daddies cannot fix.

That very day, September 9, was the moment Allie finally cried. She cried hard and deep and for a long time. She buried her head on my chest and let me hold her as we both wept. I hadn't held her that way since she was a baby. Her need for comfort ran deeper than I knew. Her behavior started to improve after that, but we still had so much more to deal with, including the funeral planned for only two days later.

The day before the funeral, Ronda and I went to the funeral home and readied Sammi's casket. Allie picked out a binkie blanket to put with Sammi. It was off-white, with a little bear head sewn into the center. The binkie was a soft fleece on top with silk underside. I bought some purple and white silk roses to put at her feet. The funeral director came in with Sammi's body and put her in the casket. She was so kind to take some white gauze and wrap Sammi's tummy where the incision was from the pathology testing. I was upset to see how her body had changed in just that short amount of time.

However, the funeral plans did not go how we intended. It should have been on September 11, but on the tenth, I noticed a problem. I noticed something of an odor when I went to the bathroom. I went to the doctor, and she told me I had a uterine infection and needed to be admitted to the hospital again. I would need to be on antibiotics right away. So that night and for the next twenty-four hours, I was on IV antibiotics, totaling five bags of it. When I was released, I was given two very strong antibiotics to take for ten days, each to be taken twice a day, 2,000 milligrams a day total. I literally felt like I was going to die. I remember telling Jack, "I think I'm dying." I felt utterly weak, and never in my life did I feel so much like I was approaching death as I did during those ten days.

At first I thought I was just depressed over the baby and tired because of my stress, but when I went for my recheck, the doctor told me I should probably never take those medications again and my reactions were not normal. I guess I didn't care about anything at that point, not even enough to gripe about the medicine. I just felt like, *What's the point? Whatever happens, happens. What can I do about it anyway?* But that despair, that passive resignation, would soon turn into my new-found ability to relinquish control and hand it over to God.

When I tried to look to the Bible for comfort, I felt even more hopeless. Yet I knew that I needed to open my Bible and at least make an effort. I decided I would read wherever it flopped open. The book that it opened to was Job. "Job?" I burst out. Then I slammed the Bible shut. I didn't want to read Job. *What a miserable reference, Lord,* I thought. The man who lost everything worse than anyone in the history of the world. Who would want to read that during their deepest sorrow? I wasn't ready to listen to God. I was only opening my Bible out of guilt. However, I believe God had other intentions in mind. Over the next few weeks, the Lord was insistent on bringing up the book of Job to me. The more we came across it, the more I resented it. I felt angry that the Lord had made this choice again. I didn't agree with his decision.

The Lord continued to insist on bringing up the book of Job to me, and finally I decided in a huff, "All right, what is it?" I opened the book and saw the following verse.

> Then Job spoke again: "If my misery could be weighed and my troubles be put on the scales, they would outweigh all the sands of the sea. That is why I spoke impulsively. For the Almighty has struck me down with his arrows. Their poison infects my spirit. God's terrors are lined up against me. Don't I have a right to complain? Don't wild donkeys bray when they find no grass, and oxen bellow when they have no food? Don't people complain about unsalted food? Does anyone want the tasteless white of an egg? My appetite disappears when I look at it; I gag at the thought of eating it! Oh, that I might have my request, that God would grant my desire. I wish he would crush me. I wish he would reach out his hand and kill me.
>
> Job 6:1–9

I thought, *Now here is a man who understands how I feel.* Then I was willing to flip the pages, and God showed me another verse in Job.

> When Job prayed for his friends, the Lord restored his fortunes. In fact, the Lord gave him twice as much as before! So the Lord blessed Job in the second half of his life even more than in the beginning.
>
> Job 42:10, 12

After I read this verse, I thought, *Well, this makes no sense. Did you take it all away so I would ask to be restored?* I closed my Bible with this angry thought still lingering in my mind. I don't know what compelled me to open the Bible again, but this time I was not going to flop open the Old Testament. I had seen enough of Job. Here is the verse God led me to next.

> Now our knowledge is partial and incomplete, and even the gift of prophecy reveals only part of the whole picture! But when full understanding comes, these partial things will become useless. When I was a child, I spoke and thought and reasoned as a child. But when I grew up, I put away childish things. Now we see things imperfectly as in a cloudy mirror, but then we will see everything with perfect clarity. All that I know now is partial and incomplete, but then I will know everything completely, just as God now knows me completely. Three things will last forever—faith,

hope, and love—and the greatest of these is love.

1 Corinthians 13:9–13

I realized that while I'm on earth, I may never fully understand his purpose in choosing to give me two children and take them back so suddenly. Somehow, these verses gave me a little bit of peace. I asked a question, and he at least was answering. I was able to get past some of my sorrow and find more of God's healing. It was certainly not an instantaneous event, and it didn't happen all at once.

My healing has been a voyage of ups and downs, going forward and backward. At times, I was mean, critical, depressed, and hopeless, but there were also times I was positive, clear, joyous, and guided with purpose. Clarity came and went in waves. One day I was convinced that the hardest part was over; the next day I was struggling again.

Confusion engulfed my mind on most days. I was so embarrassed when I couldn't remember basic tasks. *Did I wash my hands? Did I take my vitamin? Did I feed the dog today?* Then there were the bigger issues. *Where do I stand? What is my purpose? How do I go on?* Some days I had no goals, no ambition, and no way to move forward. For years, I lived my life trying to be better, trying to be whatever was expected. Now I had no ambition to move forward at all.

When I wasn't pregnant, my life revolved around getting pregnant. I ate certain ways for it, and my thoughts were constantly in hopes of it. I went certain places, I took certain medicines, and I couldn't even clean the house without thinking about *when the baby comes.* Yet now I had to live life in a manner I never did before. I had to discover one day at a time what it was like to live without knowing or planning for the future. I had to learn how to exist right in the moment. Like Jesus said, "So don't worry about tomorrow, for tomorrow will bring its own worries. Today's trouble is enough for today" (Matthew 6:34).

At first, I had resigned to God, *Okay, you win. I control nothing. Take it. Take it all; I don't want it anymore.* It was a negative, indignant release, but it was a release still the same. Before long, I realized, *Hey, this is so much better. You keep it. I really don't want it back.* This awareness helped me more than I expected. It showed me how to do exactly what Jesus spoke about in Matthew.

> Then Jesus said, "Come to me, all of you who are weary and carry heavy burdens, and I will give you rest. Take my yoke upon you. Let me teach you, because I am humble and gentle at heart, and you will find rest for your souls. For my yoke is easy to bear, and the burden I give you is light."
>
> Matthew 11:28–30

I trusted him when he took it. I knew, once and for all, that if my life experiences had taught me anything it was: I can't control *anything* about life or death, but God controls everything. God's choices can be trusted; he can be trusted. This most important realization came from the following scripture:

"For I know the plans I have for you," says the Lord. "They are plans for good and not for disaster, to give you a future and a hope. In those days when you pray, I will listen. If you look for me wholeheartedly, you will find me. I will be found by you," says the Lord. "I will end your captivity and restore your fortunes. I will gather you out of the nations where I sent you and will bring you home again to your own land."

Jeremiah 29:11–14

I had learned to accept God's control, and with that, I had to understand God doesn't intend for these things to harm me; that was never his intent. In Genesis, Joseph was sold into slavery by his brothers because of their hatred for him. In their resentment, their evil desires sought to harm Joseph, but God turned it into something wonderful when he used Joseph to save many lives during the great famine of that time.

The funeral was moved to September 18, 2008, due to my second hospitalization, but on the seventeenth, the new miscarriage class was set to begin. I had been to the class twice already and felt unsure about returning again. Though the classes had been helpful, I was nervous about starting so soon after losing Sammi. I remember debating on whether I would even attend. I concluded, *I'll go, but I won't share.*

Of course, when the other women had finished sharing their stories, suddenly my fears melted away. The words came gushing out of me like a broken faucet. I needed to get it out. I needed to share. I can still see the expressions on their faces when I answered their question, "When did this happen?" I saw their mouths drop open and their eyes widen when my reply was, "We bury Sammi tomorrow." They sat in shock and disbelief. *How could she be here? How could she be talking to us?* I hardly knew the answer myself. Somehow, it seemed easier to not be at home, thinking about the next day's events.

CHAPTER SEVEN

The funeral was on a beautiful fall day. The trees were just starting to turn yellow and orange and red. The sky was the bluest heavenly blue I had ever seen, and the wind was blowing just enough to keep things cool. The way that the trees had grown and the leaves had fallen let the sunrays beam down just on those standing at her graveside. It truly would have made a wonderful painting or portrait. The peacefulness in the air seemed to rest easily in me. We drove up to her graveside before the funeral so we wouldn't have to worry about what to expect when we arrived after the church service.

As I looked out at the readied grave, it suddenly occurred to me, *Sammi is going to be buried next to the same little boy that I attended the memorial service of weeks ago.* Little did I know, just a few weeks before, I was standing in the very spot where my own child would be buried. Somehow I felt so very connected to that little baby boy and his family. Our kids' bodies lay right next to each other on earth, and I wondered if their little spirits danced together in heaven.

As we drove by, Allie said, "I'm so excited!" I asked her why. "I'm going to see Sammi today!"

I felt a disgusting lump in my throat and a tightening in my chest as I reminded her of all we had discussed. "Yes, we are burying Sammi, but we won't be able to see her in her casket."

"But why, Momma?" I tried to explain, but nothing would ever make this easier for any of us. At the church, Allie was insistent on helping me put the baby blanket on top of Sammi's casket, and she wanted to be the one to put the teddy bear on there as well. I was glad she was so willing to be a part of the service, and I could see that she needed to be included.

Many of our friends came, also the moms' group from church. They all came to offer support and encouragement. Before we started the service, Allie hid in the corner of the church. I had to reassure her that it was okay so she would come sit by me.

During the service, the pastor read from many texts, including from the book of Job. I looked over at Jack and widened my eyes. "Can you believe this? What is it with Job?" When the funeral service was over, Jack walked to the front of the sanctuary and picked up Sammi's tiny little casket. My quilt remained there as the covering, and we quietly followed Jack to the funeral director's car. When we arrived at the cemetery, Jack placed her casket on her grave. After the pastor finished his prayers, I asked Ronda to do a few readings. Included were the verses Mark 9:36–37 and Mark 10:14.

When all of the prayers were over, there was an awkward silence. No one quite knew what to do, and no one moved. So I walked over to her casket and picked up the quilt; then I immediately grabbed on to Jack overflowing with tears. He didn't seem to be holding me very tightly; he was more in a state of shock. Allie saw me crying and burst into tears, holding on to my leg. I dropped to my knees and held her close. "Momma's okay, baby. Remember, tears help me heal. Tears get out the hurting, remember?"

Moments later, when everyone was saying their good-byes to us, Allie wandered off to the cars and was walking around the grass in circles alone. The pastor went over to see about her, but she walked away from him. I excused myself and walked toward her, and then she ran to me.

"What are you doing, baby? Mommy's okay. I love you." She squeezed my neck. With that reassurance, she started dancing in circles, content to be alone. I gave her some space and finished saying good-bye. When it was time to go, Jack grabbed the flower planter that a friend of ours brought as a gift from his parents, and I grabbed the remaining flowers. I was ready to be home and for this day to be over.

Jack was on a family medical leave that would end in nearly two weeks. I told him that I really wanted to get away. So while he was still on his leave, we planned a trip to go away for a few days to the North Shore (northern Minnesota). We planned our trip, taking a special detour for Allie to go horseback riding. We found a ranch online that offered a great deal. When we arrived, the owner took Allie and me on a four-wheeler, along with her German shepherd, Haley, to round up her horses. There were over a hundred, and the experience was one of a lifetime. I can still hear her voice, "Hup! Hup! Hup!" as the horses ran to the stable. For the horses that didn't cooperate, Haley nipped at their tails, barking and sending them running. I had never seen horses run like that before; it was truly breathtaking.

The horseback ride was so relaxing. Granted, it was not the best decision, considering I was still healing from the infection in my uterus. I was quite sore that whole afternoon, but the next stop was an indoor water park. Allie and Jack had a great time while I relaxed in the room. The final stop was at a lakeside resort. I had never seen such a beautiful place as this, and I was so happy to be there. There is something about being in nature that is very healing. It put us closer to God, through his creation, and away from the distractions of this busy world. However, I noticed that in this silence I was all too aware of the empty feelings that had begun to consume me.

I spent most of the weekend debating with God and trying to start an argument with Jack to express my own anger, confusion, and resentments. I was frustrated that Jack didn't seem to understand. I was convinced that he couldn't understand, but I was wrong. Since I spent so much time thinking about how isolated *I* was and how alone *I* felt, I had completely disregarded Jack's sorrow.

Jack is a very tolerant person and the most generous, caring soul I have ever known, but even he can be pushed to his limits. In frustration, he finally told me, "You know, you weren't the only one who lost Sammi. I had dreams of life with her too. The only time I got to hold my little girl was from the church to her grave."

It broke my heart to see him suffering this way. He told me about some of his expectations that were lost when she died, and I began to realize that I didn't want to let Jack or Allie feel pain. I wanted to protect them from it, so I refused to acknowledge what they were going through. Nevertheless, I soon started to resent the fact that Jack didn't seem to have the same sorrows as I did. Truthfully, he was hurting. Only I didn't want to see it, and he didn't want to add to my worries by showing it.

What a miserable battle we fought, simply to end with the discovery that we were only hurting each other more by not being honest about our pain. Even if it seemed like the right way to prevent hurting one other, it only caused us more sorrow in the end. Jack had always been my rock, my safe place. But if that trip was for any purpose, it helped me realize that even my rock has needs.

During that month after Sammi's funeral, the doctor called me with some long awaited news. The testing showed that our Sammi was healthy. There was nothing physically wrong with her. However, her placenta was full of blood clots. Due to the fact that I had preeclampsia with Allie's birth, plus the two miscarriages, one with confirmed blood clots in Sammi's placenta, they were concerned I had Antiphospholipid Syndrome (a blood clotting disease). I was later tested for this disease but showed negative. My new gynecologist said that despite my results she would treat me as if I did have the disease, considering I had all the typical symptoms. For future reference, I was to take a single baby aspirin every day starting from before conception.

Jack and I felt torn about the idea of trying to get pregnant again. What if this happened again? How would it affect Allie to endure another loss? We talked about it, but we didn't feel it was even realistic that we could get pregnant, considering it took four years to conceive our last pregnancy. We didn't begin trying, but we weren't preventing either.

When we first came home from the hospital, after Sammi's delivery, I hesitated to keep any of her things. At first I wanted to bury it all with her. I felt like I wanted to bury the entire period of my life and never face it again. Yet something in me caused me to keep her journal. I picked it up and read it for a while, crying as I realized how empty my words would be. But then I decided to create one final entry.

> October 12, 2008 (One month, one week past your delivery)
> So you were a girl. I feel sick writing in here, knowing how the last entry was made while you were still inside me. I'm devastated because this note to you is not going to be read when you have your first pregnancy. I'm nauseous thinking about how these words are just empty words to you in heaven. My hopes in your life and what you would be are all gone. You're onto a different plane now. You've moved on to heaven, working and growing in the Lord. I desperately am sorry that I didn't know how to save you.
>
> I'm heartbroken, Lord. Another baby gone to you. How my soul aches for my Samantha Grace to still be here. I feel horrid that all it might have taken was a single baby aspirin to save my two babies' lives. What has my body done? Why have you given me this disease that makes me form clots that only end in aborting my babies? My love for you

and for my babies surely must outweigh the need for the lesson in this loss. I'm sorry, Lord; I don't mean to presume that your plan is meaningless. I'm devastated, confused, and utterly heartbroken. My soul hurts so deeply that it retches within me. Please, heal my core. Please, give me back the one way I needed to heal. Help me, Lord. I will come, Lord. I have. I'm here now, begging for healing and hope. Don't even guide me. I don't care about tomorrow. Just give me today, meet me here today, help me heal. It hurts, God. It hurts! It hurts! Heal me. Help me, Lord. Hope, Lord. Hope, Lord. I need hope.

I love you, Samantha Grace. You're in my heart.

CHAPTER EIGHT

For weeks, I returned to the Bible study, going through chapter after chapter, then returning to the group to gather and share thoughts about each lesson and the spiritual realizations that God had brought into our lives as a result of those lessons. The first meeting had somehow deposited onto me an invisible pressure to keep up appearances as being spiritually strong. I felt the need to be an example of God's strength and to prove the peace I felt during this horrible experience was real. By week four, however, I realized that my need for the support of the class weighed heavier than my pride. My façade of being strong ripped open as I revealed my struggle to deal with this one-month marker of my loss and everyone else's expectations that seemed to pressure me to "get over it by now." The group completely understood my position and offered me great support and advice in dealing with these issues.

A few weeks into our Bible study, we were discussing the concept of memories and their effects on our spiritual lives; that week, I went home filled with inspiration. I wondered, *What other ways have Satan's lies affected my life?* I thought about my darkest memories, the ones that haunt me the most, and I realized, *The God I love would never have left me alone in those situations, so why is it that when I remember it I feel so alone?* I wanted to change those memories. I wanted to see the truth where Satan had planted a lie.

Here began another time in my life that when I became ready and willing, God moved me forward. I began with this prayer:

> Lord, I ask that you please reveal to me one memory at a time so I can see where you were in that memory. I pray that you would use this time, this moment of recollection, to heal the bad feelings that for years I have associated with each of these memories. In healing these, I know you will take the power away from the memory so it no longer can be a hindrance or a vulnerability to my walk with you. Heal my heart, and take my hand, Lord, as I try to bring total openness to your holy presence into every aspect of my being. I want to learn to see you as you really were in each memory so I can learn to see you with me as a constant now. I ask that this be healing in my home, my heart, and in my future. I pray this in Jesus' name, amen.

When I began writing in the journal, I started with the most haunting memory of my childhood. The memory of this event ran constantly through my mind and seemed to be Satan's greatest weapon against my feelings toward God as well as my interpretation of where God is during the hardest moments of my life.

The old memory is revealed: I'm ten years old. My mother just died. There is a cloud of uncertainty and confusion that seems to have swallowed up my once predictable existence. The house is swarming with people. I know some of them, but mostly there are many strangers. I wander outside. There are boys of all ages playing basketball in our driveway. *Who are they?* I wonder. I sit down on the cold, hard concrete steps. My bare feet feel how smooth the steps are.

I am alone. No one seems to notice me. My hurt feels more like numbness and shock. The door opens and shuts as unknown people rush in and out. No one sees me. I am lost in my own home. I watch the driveway, expecting the boys to move out of the way; I know at any minute my parents will drive up and rescue me. I don't feel safe. I wait. I wait. I tire of waiting. They never come. I go inside as the darkness of evening arrives, and my fear outweighs my hope. Alone, all alone. I'm homesick. *Where is Momma? I want my momma.*

The new memory is healed: I'm coming outside after feeling the call of someone, a familiar voice. I sit down, feeling relief from the warm, humid August air on the coolness of the concrete steps. I lean my elbow on someone's knee. I look up and see Jesus' face. He tilts his head slightly and gives me a gentle chin-up smile. His arm reaches around me and pulls my shoulder in closer. I smile and lean my head into his chest. I am not alone. His arms are strong and safe. We wait for Momma together. He knows I will see her again, and I believe him.

I went back to the Bible study group and shared with them how this memory didn't feel so heavy and dark anymore. In fact, it hasn't even returned to my mind since being healed; Satan lost his power in it. I was able to ask and receive an answer to the question, "Where would Jesus have been during that dark moment of my life?" Now, for all the rest of my life, the power of that negative memory has been disabled by the truth of God's love. They seemed genuinely interested in this memory-changing technique, and several of the women used it themselves to heal their own difficult memories.

We discussed how Satan's lies, within our thoughts, are the single, most destructive weapon he has. I won't allow him to have the power over my memories anymore. I wouldn't allow him the control over my thoughts. It became my goal to know the absolute truth from God in every area of my mind and spirit. I knew the only way to find this was to read his Word and fill my thoughts with positive truths. Focusing on bad memories, gripes, and complaints and pettiness was not from God. I also realized that I couldn't allow Satan to lie to me about my miscarriage. I had to look for God's truth.

This led me to the realization that my life had been altered. Whether I wanted it to be different or not, I had no choice. It was forever changed, and if

I did not start filling that hole with something positive, then the negatives would take over and bring me to destruction. Jesus says this about the devil: "He was a murderer from the beginning. He has always hated the truth, because there is no truth in him. When he lies, it is consistent with his character; for he is a liar and the father of lies" (John 8:44b). How else would I expect to battle the devil's lies, except in the one place that he most effectively separated me from God—my thoughts? If one of Satan's lies such as, "This isn't fair," would be allowed to linger long enough, it would multiply and allow for more lies such as, "It's because God doesn't love you." One small thought that is not from God cannot be allowed to linger, or else it will rapidly morph into the most destructive force in my mind.

I knew the reason I felt so lost in the beginning of my healing was because I was thrown instantaneously into a completely new way of thinking and a new way to look at life. Nothing else around me had changed; only my life had changed.

During that time, when well-meaning friends told me how I was "lucky" and that my baby was "probably better off" or that I could "always have more children," I literally wanted to explode. If their husband had died, would they accept a comment that he was better off dead than alive, and not to worry, they could always get another one? Who could replace the life of another in value? No one but God.

These comments made me feel so out of place with all of my friends. It became a silent awkwardness. I wasn't sure if it was simply my own feelings of being on the outside or if they were acting differently toward me. Perhaps it was a little of both. Either way, I found it very difficult to connect with those that I once could easily relate to. Everything became very serious for me, and all the little daily complaints seemed so insignificant in the scope of my life since it had changed. I couldn't talk the same way; I couldn't think the same way. I was in a state of total disarray.

During those most vulnerable times, Satan attacked me the hardest, but these attacks were not always obvious. Sometimes these attacks were very subtle and happened inside my mind as a part of a spiritual battle, a battle that required me to *choose* to win. The Lord showed me I couldn't win any battle by standing still in the middle of it. I had to be moved into action! My miscarriage left me feeling out of place, but I had no choice except to find a way to move forward. I couldn't stand by and watch the rest of my family life crumble to pieces over my deep sorrow.

I realized that if I was not acting and thinking *for* God then I was automatically *against* him. There was no middle ground, no in-between, no way of lying low or remaining neutral in this world. The Lord says, "I know all the things you do, that you are neither hot nor cold. I wish that you were one or the other! But since you are like lukewarm water, neither hot nor cold, I will spit you out of my mouth!" (Revelation 3:15–16). He also says this:

> I correct and discipline everyone I love. So be diligent and turn from your indifference. Look! I stand at the door and knock. If you hear my voice and open the door, I will come in, and we will share a meal together as friends. Those who are victorious will sit with me on my throne, just as I was victorious and sat with my Father on his throne.

When I read this, I felt determination. I thought, *I have to choose. I choose to see any sorrow as the Lord's fire, purifying me to holiness, as gold is purified. I can no longer be on the neutral ground.* In fact, I could no longer even think in the same way as before; my entire process of thought had been altered. "Don't copy the behavior and customs of this world, but let God transform you into a new person by changing the way you think. Then you will learn to know God's will for you, which is good and pleasing and perfect" (Romans 12:2). I knew I had to make the most of our tragedy; I had to let it change me or else the sorrow might consume me. I wasn't sure how I would do it, but I had to find a way to fulfill the purpose of miscarriages in my life.

CHAPTER NINE

Finally the time came for the Bible study to end, and it was time for the memorial service. There was no avoiding it this time. I had to remember Elizabeth and Sammi, and I had to let go of them both. I let go of the pew and walked nervously to the front of the church. As I stood at the altar, trembling with my letter in hand, I read:

Dear heaven,

I've got a lot to say to you today. As a whole, you have collected from me four of the most important people in my life: my mother and father, two of my three daughters, and not to mention the countless others whom I have loved and lost. There are things that I wanted to say to them, things that I imagined doing with them, and people that are in my life now that I really wanted them to meet. From time to time, I have blamed you for robbing me of that chance. I often looked at my life and asked you, *Why?* I never understood how you could take so many people out of my life. When you took them, there was nothing but silence left here with me, and it was a silence that hurt. I hate the quiet.

Heaven, I used to wonder if you would ever want me. There was a time that I thought you must *not* want me but that you just wanted to *punish* me by filling my life with that awful deafening silence, as you took those that I loved away from me one by one. Yet, even in the silence, I often strained my ears in the hopes of hearing them. Sometimes I would pretend that they were still here with me. I knew that if I could just hear them, then I wouldn't have to face another day in silence without them.

One day when I was listening for them, I got frustrated waiting to hear something and decided to make my own noise. It didn't quite fill the emptiness, but it wasn't nearly as silent. I busied myself with every kind of bustle in order to fill that unpleasant void left by their silence. Eventually, I gave up that tiresome lifestyle. I realized that even the replacement voices were not nearly as good as the voices I had lost, and I didn't want the substitutes anymore—I wanted the real voices!

At that point, I began to grow very angry. I collapsed on the floor of my quiet, empty world and stopped being quiet myself. I screamed! I screamed, cried, and yelled at you! "How could you make me endure this silence?" When I finished my rant, I decided that I was not going to listen to you anymore. I was wrapped up in my own sorrow. Yet, in that moment, I thought that I heard something. I stopped my fit long enough to listen, and there was nothing but silence. Disgusted at your trickery, I quit listening, and again, there it was: a noise! I realized that I *was* hearing something but not with my outward ears; it was a kind of spiritual inner ear. When I tried to listen with those ears, I *could* hear! Finally I found a way to listen to you.

Ah, the healing; the wholeness. It was as wonderful as opening a window to a cool breeze on a warm day. I felt its mysterious arms wrap me up. It was all right there, everywhere, all around me. How could I live my life without knowing you were so close, practically inside me? *Wait!* I realized. *You were inside me!* Heaven, I found you. I found you here, in my heart, in my soul, in my mind, everywhere in and all around me!

Best of all, I could hear them, my family. Their voices were vague, but I could truly hear them! I could feel them in you. I could sense them. Suddenly, you opened that window a little wider to me. You let me see inside you, heaven. When I looked, I saw Momma first. I saw her holding a little girl. She was standing beneath a grand oak tree. The sky was blue, and the grass was yellow and green. Momma laughed as she spun the little girl around and around. Then I blinked. Beside her, I could see another little girl. It was Elizabeth! Her long, black, curly hair bounced as she jumped excitedly, clapping her hands. She laughed with giddy delight as Momma held the baby's tiny hand and spun her around. The baby was Samantha! Sammi smiled and laughed, and her head flung back in pure joy, ringlets flailing in the wind.

Heaven, I know you heard me when I called out to them, "Momma! Momma!" Yet their laughter was too loud, and with it, they couldn't hear me. I laughed and cried in joy at the sight of them. Momma put her hands in the air and waved them around as Elizabeth copied her movements. They danced and bounced and played. Elizabeth was a ball full of energy as she jumped onto a swing hanging from the branch of the tree and took off running to get it going full speed. I just stood there silent, watching through your window.

My mind wondered back to the heaviness of the world I had been living in, and I thought to myself, *They deserve this place. They deserve this everlasting joy. They deserve to play and laugh and be filled with love for all eternity. They deserve to bring God joy this way, and they need this, to be wrapped in his love.*

I felt a little guilty wanting to take it from them. I couldn't ask them to leave that place. I couldn't ask them to come back with me, but now I *could* look forward to going to them, as King David said of his own son. The entirety of the joy and the fullness of that place still astounded me. I stood only at the window, but the wholeness of that place was so overwhelming that I could not withhold my tears of awe-inspired joy.

I smiled as I opened my outward eyes, and I could see that this silence was only a closed window between me and the ones I loved. I felt comforted to know their joy was so beyond what was possible to feel here. Heaven, I realize that you didn't punish me. You have *rewarded* them! You've blessed them so beyond what I could ever have imagined.

So thank you.
Sincerely, from Earth

After reading my letter, I finished by saying these words, "I know that my glimpse through heaven's window was merely a way that God was able to help me understand what ultimate peace in him can be. But in that moment, I realized that the silence I once felt has now become stillness. The emptiness I felt *before* is now exceedingly full of God's Holy Spirit. There is no longer barrenness in my soul. I could have left that hole unfilled and sat my entire life staring at that emptiness, angry at it, filling it with earthly business. But I didn't. I let God in, and he filled it up with something that could help me, something positive that could change my life. When I think about that old empty spot in my life, I wonder, *What room would I have made for God otherwise?* He moved them into a wonderful place so that *he* could move into their place in my life. I would want for nothing else now."

Thank you, Lord, for moving into the emptiness that otherwise might have destroyed me. Thank you for letting me see you and for healing me. Their deaths cut deep into my heart, but that wound allowed you to heal me deeper than I could have ever foreseen. So I give this all to you. Amen.

Without making eye contact, I walked quietly back to my seat. The other mothers took their turns to share tributes for their children. We tearfully embraced each memorial, understanding on the deepest levels how precious our little ones were and still are to us, and how devastating their losses had been to our individual lives and families. Even more so, we knew how necessary our healing has been for a healthy survival of these losses. I found that by offering strength and support to others I actually had received it tenfold onto myself.

When the service came to a close, the director gave me an opportunity to present my gifts to the women. I walked behind the far left pew and picked up one of the gift bags. As I hugged this mom and gave this gift, I heard myself whisper the words, "I love you." Only, it wasn't me saying this, it was God saying this through me. In my mind, I didn't know these women well enough to love them. Yet, in my heart, I did.

Each mother received their gift of a memorial quilt. Each was specially designed as a tribute to their lost babies. Some of the design concepts I collected during our previous meetings. A few of the ideas I included just because, and those little additions were somehow the most noteworthy. They asked me how I could have known the significance of these items in their personal lives, things they had never shared during group, and all I could say was, "I didn't know that about you. But God knows you. And he must have made me choose that." We all stepped out into a reception hall, where we were able to share about our experiences with the baby dolls. I was embarrassed to say that I had let mine sit on top of our computer desk for the entire week.

During the reception, I was surprised by the feelings of sorrow that swept over me as I thought about this being our last meeting. However, saying good-bye to these women seemed to be a sorrow in and of itself for me. How could I have shared such intimate details of my grief with them and then just walk away, unsure of whether I would ever see them again? I knew that God had brought this group of women together for his reasoning and that we were able to serve a special purpose in each other's seasons of grieving. Now we each had to move forward alone into our new season. I wouldn't be able to stay in the grief any longer, and I realized what I truly feared was the unknown changes ahead. So in a bittersweet good-bye, we hugged and waved, and I silently promised within myself never to forget what God had done for us when we came together once a week for those two months. Even though we had finished our gatherings, we knew that in our hearts and spirits we would be connected for life through the lives of our children in heaven.

CHAPTER TEN

Little did I know there would be even more hurdles ahead for our family. When my in-laws left in November, I could still feel the numbness of my grief lurking beneath the surface. The shock of what I had just been though had finally begun to wear off. My initial burst of sorrow had been expressed, and now I was entering into a new process: learning to live with our loss.

Despite the fragility of my heart, I carried myself with a newfound strength in God. I found a place where the opinions of others meant nothing to me. I realized that their opinions could never be relevant if they had not walked in my shoes. I never felt so free and connected to God in all my life as I did during that time, just after we lost our Sammi. However, the high did not last very long. As brave as I felt, as courageous as I was convinced I had become, I was not prepared for the months ahead. Here we were in mid-November, facing the holidays.

Everyone around us chatted about what their holiday plans were. They asked us how would we

spend the holidays, and I smiled and said, "At home."
When really what I wanted to say was, *What do you
think? Our family is 1,200 miles away! We'll be sitting at
home depressed thinking about the baby we just buried last
month!* I still felt angry at their apparent insensitivities
to our loss. Did they really think we had just moved on
and forgotten what had just happened? But they were
not trying to hurt me. Just trying to make conversa-
tion really, but I resented that everyone else's life could
move on as if nothing had ever happened, because mine
couldn't. I didn't like the pressure to conform.

I have to admit that first Christmas was a difficult one. It was only three months after we delivered
Sammi, and we expected it to be tough. For as long as
I can remember, Christmas had always been my favorite time of year. I always started looking forward to
the holidays as early as each September beforehand. I
just loved it. A time of cooking and laughing, sharing
love and thoughtfulness through gifts, and remembering the good times with people I loved. I looked forward to making my gifts personal and sincere; it was
my favorite part of Christmas. Nevertheless, this year
was very different.

Nearly two weeks before Christmas, I started dread-
ing the whole season. If it had not been for Allie, I'm
certain we would have skipped Christmas altogether. I
told Jack, "It feels impossible to get into the Christmas
spirit." He smiled and nodded in agreement; I knew
he understood. After all the talks we had during my
pregnancy for Sammi about how I would be "big and
pregnant" for Christmas, it was depressing just to think
of the season being so barren. To make matters even
more difficult to face, I noticed that Allie was missing
Sammi as well.

One morning, a couple weeks before Christmas, she told me something really odd. "Mommy, you have a baby in your tummy." I could not for the life of me figure out why she was saying such a thing.

I asked her, "What makes you think that?"

"I just know."

Of course, I was not satisfied with that, so I asked her, "How do you know?"

"Well, my brain told me so!" She said it in such a matter-of-fact tone. I just smiled and explained to her that mommy did not have a baby in her tummy. I just assumed she was missing Sammi and tried to focus on making Christmas as normal as possible.

Before long, I began to notice every baby reminder as a direct link to the expectation of how pregnant I would have been by that point. Ronda, hoping to lift my spirits, invited me to a Christmas party at her church. At the last minute, I decided to go with her, hoping to take my mind off of things. When we arrived, there seemed to be an abundance of pregnant women. Not only were they pregnant, but they were as pregnant as I *would* have been.

The speaker's message seemed to be yet another blow to my heart, as she talked about how Jesus' mother, Mary, must have felt being pregnant, illustrating her point with a photo slide show documenting her own personal pregnancy growth from twelve weeks until forty. I felt disgusted. As if my pain weren't enough to deal with, I was forced to face pregnant women every-where! I didn't know if it was a direct sign from God or just my obsession getting more severe. Either way I was too embarrassed to admit to anyone how inces-santly my thoughts kept running back to life "before" my loss. For months that was all of what defined my life. Everything that happened was referred to as either *before* or *after* Sammi died.

Just before Christmas, I was due for my period, but I was not having any of the usual signs. I began wondering if I was pregnant. As soon as the thought entered my mind, I brushed it off. *Gimme a break. As if you could be pregnant. You tried four years to conceive Sammi; do you honestly think three months later you're pregnant again?* I reminded myself about all the times that I took pregnancy tests, with as much hope as desperation, and how many times they were negative. I, as a woman who frantically wanted a baby, was often fooled by my own body into thinking I was pregnant when I really was not. During my infertility, it was all I thought about, but after having lost a child, I was surprised to find myself enduring a false pregnancy so soon.

I remember talking to Jack about it, crying, "It's hard enough facing Christmas without her, but now to have a false pregnancy." By this point, I was in a deep pool of self-pity, and I could feel myself beginning to drown in it. The strength I felt in God started to unravel, and as the frustration heightened, every feeling that I had been bottling up just started to erupt. I needed to prove to myself that I was not pregnant, or else I would never be able to move on. I took three at-home pregnancy tests, and they all said negative. Did I believe them? No. I needed more proof.

Next, I called the doctor's office and told the nurse that I felt like I could be pregnant, the test said negative, and my period wasn't here yet (granted it wasn't *late* either). She said, "Well, you can come in, but if it's negative, you might just need to wait another week and take another test." I made an appointment for December 24.

The doctor gave me a blood test to determine the level of pregnancy hormone, and it said <0.01, which indicated nothing. They require it to be seven before they consider you to be pregnant. She told me to come back in a few days if I had not gotten my period. So, on December 26, 2008, I took another blood test. This time the number was six. She smiled. "Well, that is a good sign. Maybe."

"What do you mean? You know, I have to go out there and tell my husband whether or not I'm pregnant. What am I supposed to tell him, *maybe*?" I was puzzled but hopeful. This time I had a good sign to hang on to.

"I'm telling you there is a good chance. Your number has tripled in just a couple days. Let's give it until January 2. We'll do another test then." I felt somewhat bewildered. What was I supposed to feel? Happy? Scared? I couldn't truly feel anything definite until the next blood test. It seemed like I would have to wait years to know the truth.

During this time of waiting, I was desperate for answers. I flipped open my Bible one day, and it opened to a book called 1 Samuel. I thought, *Oh, that's neat. I didn't know there was even a book in the Bible called Samuel.* I read the first chapter and couldn't believe what I was seeing! Here was a woman who could truly understand my sorrows. She so desperately wanted a child. She knew of the harsh judgments of others as she struggled with her barrenness. She prayed to God, asking for a child, and he heard her prayer. Was this God's confirmation to me that we would indeed have a child? I knew right then that if we had a son, his name must be Samuel. It was clearly a sign from God.

> And though he loved Hannah, he would give her only one choice portion because the Lord had given her no children. So Peninnah would taunt Hannah and make fun of her because the Lord had kept her from having children. Year after year it was the same—Peninnah would taunt Hannah as they went to the Tabernacle. Each time, Hannah would be reduced to tears and would not even eat. Hannah was in deep anguish, crying bitterly as she prayed to the Lord. And she made this vow: "O Lord of Heaven's Armies, if you will look upon my sorrow and answer my prayer and give me a son, then I will give him back to you. He will be yours for his entire lifetime, and as a sign that he has been dedicated to the Lord, his hair will never be cut." And in due time she gave birth to a son. She named him Samuel, for she said, "I asked the Lord for him."

> 1 Samuel 1:5–7, 10–11, 20

Eventually, despite the tortuously long wait, we did go back, and on the drive there, I reread the chapter in 1 Samuel out loud to Jack. This time the doctor said my hormone number was 486. She told me, "Well, you are definitely pregnant." At first I was taken aback. *Are you kidding me?* I didn't know how to feel: thankful or terrified. I wanted this baby, but would it survive? Would I survive? Even more surprising was that Allie turned out to be right! I actually *was* pregnant when she told me there was a baby in my tummy.

I came home in utter shock. We had warned his parents after Christmas that we might be pregnant again, and we would let them know more after this next test. It was more of a warning than a spreading of joyous news. We weren't sure how they would handle the news. I had only *just* lost Samantha. It was so soon. It truly defied all odds. But I just hoped in my heart that this was really our miracle.

They were happy to hear the news and were being very hopeful with us. Though the idea of being pregnant was wonderful, since we had at least gotten that far, the concept of surviving the pregnancy was terrifying. I had a million questions running through my mind: *Will this baby make it? How far will the pregnancy go if it doesn't? When do we tell everyone? How do we tell them? How will Allie take the news? Are we prepared to deal with the same physical and emotional horrors of loss again?* It was all completely out of our hands. What could we do? Nothing but wait.

We told a few close friends, and I quickly realized that I didn't want people to be too happy about it. I wanted them to be pleased, but softly. I could hear the relief in their voices as their thoughts seemed to slap me in the face. *At least now she has this one to replace the last one. Maybe now she won't be sad anymore. Maybe she'll forget, and then we can forget too!* I resented any thrilled response. My tender spot for Samantha did not harden with another child. This baby was not Samantha all over again. This was a whole new kid, with a whole new life, and though new joy can be a comfort to old pain, it can never heal or replace.

Here again was a time that I felt my friends no longer could relate to me. I felt angry that we could not seem to connect. It was as if someone had taken away who I was, and I was suddenly a stranger again. They didn't understand me, and I barely understood myself. I longed for the feelings of security that I felt when I connected so strongly to God. Here is a journal entry from that time:

> I'm so sick of everyone expecting that old Kristie to return, as if I am no longer good enough, as if my grief is not truly worth lasting this long or changing me. I hate that I teeter-totter between the image of the old me and the person I know I am now. I'm ready to walk away from these people who knew me before Sammi died and move on to people who have yet to meet me. Then at least the expectation of me changing is no longer there.
>
> Get me out of the old. Get me on to the new. It's the most lost feeling. You no longer belong in the world you had settled so snuggly into. You are a member of a hidden society, unwillingly forced to become a member of the terrible club of mothers who have lost babies during pregnancy.
>
> I hate their relief at my new pregnancy. I despise their hopeful glances that maybe this will get me back to how they felt comfortable with me. I hate that my sorrow changing me is so unacceptable in their eyes. I want it to change me; I want it to make me new again. I cannot stop myself from being different. I cannot stop myself or change my past. I can't be anyone but me. My life cir-

cumstances have made me this way, and I will not hide it for anyone. No one is worth living a lie for. No one!

This pregnancy was going to be a long haul, and I knew it right away. I started analyzing every emotion, every thought, and every premonition. I compared every twinge or lack of twinge to the previous pregnancy loss. *Was this what happened before?* I have to admit that the fear of loss that engulfed me with Samantha didn't seem remotely close to the fears I had now. I *knew* exactly what could happen this time. I knew what devastation it was to lose a baby at eight weeks, and I knew what torture it was to deliver, bury, and mourn a baby at eighteen and a half weeks. I was afraid, to say the least.

A couple of months into this pregnancy, I started feeling even more worried. Technically, I was only eight weeks, but for some reason I had a new fear beginning to take over. *Why am I not showing yet? I should be so much further along by now!* I didn't understand my own thoughts. Why did I worry so much about showing? I wasn't far enough along; it was crazy to be feeling desperate to show.

Suddenly, the truth occurred to me in a blinding flash of insight. Somewhere in the back of my mind, I was combining my pregnancies. I lost my Samantha in September, just a week and a half shy of my halfway point. I was pregnant again in December, and by the end of January, we were quickly approaching what would have been Samantha's due date. My pregnancies were overlapping. It is the most surreal experience to be pregnant a second time during what would have been the end of your last pregnancy. It was all very confusing to my body and mind. I was not finished being pregnant the full nine months of the last one. Yet here I was starting over again.

Once we passed Samantha's due date, I finally started to relax a bit. I felt some sense of release and was able to separate the two pregnancies more easily. I was very grateful to be pregnant again so soon. I knew that if this pregnancy made it, if this child survived, then I would know for the rest of that child's life that it would not have existed had our Samantha made it. It would have been impossible to have created this child had I still been pregnant with Sammi, so it was our miracle. Well, I hoped it would be.

For the first part of my pregnancy, I went to the doctor almost on a weekly basis. The longest I went between appointments for the first trimester was two weeks at a time. My new doctor was the best doctor I had ever seen in my life. She was so compassionate, so gentle with my paranoia. She made me feel it was okay to be worried, and if I ever got too worried, I could easily come in and she would check on things. She kept her word too. I came in so often. I was embarrassed at my numerous trips, but I didn't care enough not to get checked.

I can remember one ultrasound. Jack and I had been arguing. We were stressed to the limit as we both struggled to keep our fears and anxieties under control. Jack had become the main caretaker of me, our daughter, and our home for nearly a year. From the previous April through the end of September, I was so sick: sick during my pregnancy, sick recovering from losing the pregnancy, sick during the first trimester of this new pregnancy. Aside from the fact that it was more than he could take to see me so sick all of the time, he was also dealing with his own fears about this new pregnancy and what we might go through.

We went in for the doctor's appointment, and my blood pressure was high. I did all I could to keep from bursting into tears as we both sat silent in our anger. The doctor came in, and during the ultrasound, the baby moved. I looked at Jack and finally spoke. It was the first words I had spoken to him in hours. "Did you see that?" He nodded but was in too much shock to say a word. When the doctor gave me the ultrasound picture, I burst into tears. "We just ... really ... needed to see that." She put her hand comfortingly on my shoulder.

As we walked out of the office that day, I could just feel Jack's relief. He apologized for being so angry, and we both cried as we sat in the car thinking about how we never got to see Samantha move on her ultrasounds. Just seeing that one move made us feel so connected to this new baby. The next couple of ultrasounds were amazing as we watched the baby move and bounce around and steadily grow. Finally, at fourteen weeks, I was able to hear the baby's heartbeat on the monitor. It was music to my ears and comfort to my soul.

Every day dragged on like a week. Every week seemed to be months in the making. I worried I would never get there. However, my fears intensified even more as I approached a critical anniversary that no one on earth seemed to recognize but me. I hit sixteen weeks. It was unable to be confirmed whether Samantha had died at sixteen and a half weeks or seventeen weeks. I delivered her at eighteen and a half weeks, so from the time that I reached this milestone in my new pregnancy until my next ultrasound, I was a total mess. I was frantic with anxiety going to the doctor's office twice a week.

I developed anxiety-induced hives at the end of my seventeenth week. When I walked into urgent care that day, I was just sick inside as I waited to hear if the baby still had a heartbeat. I had no real reason to worry. I had no pain, no bleeding, just my own vulnerabilities in my mind.

The doctor walked in, and I burst into tears. I didn't stop crying for about fifteen minutes. I kept saying how embarrassed I was that I was crying and how I didn't even know why, but in my mind I was saying, *It's because you're scared; just say it, you're scared.* Thanks to the doctors at the Mayo Clinic for giving me the time, patience, and comfort of knowing that there are many patients like me that have suffered loss and in their subsequent pregnancies been just as paranoid and anxiety-ridden as me. I think it's important for others to know that they are not alone in how they feel.

Even though this time was one of my most trying, I also had one of my biggest turnarounds then as well. I remember that at sixteen weeks a lady passed in front of me during church with a little girl who was the age that Samantha would have been, and I burst into tears at the sight of her. *God,* I wondered, *does she know how blessed she is to have that baby? Or is she taking her for granted the way we did with Allie before our losses?*

A week and a half later, I went to visit an old friend, the mother of the little baby boy buried next to Sammi. She had just delivered a healthy baby girl. As I found myself holding this tiny baby girl, I was filled with hope. It occurred to me that I really could be holding my own baby in just a few months, and that maybe, just maybe, I would have that opportunity to love and hold an infant child of my own again. As we celebrated the birth of their beautiful miracle baby and marveled at the bravery in their demeanor as her husband prepared to leave for Iraq, I finally felt hopeful that our child could make it as well. They offered me hope just by being who they are. I could face today, tomorrow, and the many months ahead.

However, much to Jack's disappointment, this meeting did not remove *all* of my anxiety. So as a result of one of my late night crying spells, Jack decided he was going to find a heart monitor that we could use at home, and he found one online for less than $100. If you could figure out the costs of what we spent in emergency room visits and add it to the amount of doctor's visits during my panic attacks, the heart monitor saved us a ton of money. At eighteen and a half weeks, the heart monitor arrived, just in time for my first ultrasound in almost two months. This was the big ultrasound, the one most women get at twenty weeks. We couldn't wait to find out what the baby would be.

She is a girl, our Ruthie. Would she ever get to know how much she means to us? Would we get a chance to hold her? Jack told me that he was ready for her to be home, ready to hold her. I knew how he felt. We were scared to face the months ahead. Yet the Lord reminded me of something very important, his love and his faithfulness.

What shall we say about such wonderful things as these? If God is for us, who can ever be against us? Since he did not spare even his own Son but gave him up for us all, won't he also give us everything else? Who dares accuse us whom God has chosen for his own? No one—for God himself has given us right standing with himself. Who then will condemn us? No one—for Christ Jesus died for us and was raised to life for us, and he is sitting in the place of honor at God's right hand, pleading for us. Can anything ever separate us from Christ's love? Does it mean he no longer loves us if we have trouble or calamity, or are persecuted, or hungry, or destitute, or in danger, or threatened with death? (As the Scriptures say, "For your sake we are killed every day; we are being slaughtered like sheep.") No, despite all these things, overwhelming victory is ours through Christ, who loved us. And I am convinced that nothing can ever separate us from God's love. Neither death nor life, neither angels nor demons, neither our fears for today nor our worries about tomorrow—not even the powers of hell can separate us from God's love. No power in the sky above or in the earth below—indeed, nothing in all creation will ever be able to separate us from the love of God that is revealed in Christ Jesus our Lord.

Romans 8:31–39

CHAPTER ELEVEN

When I looked back on my miscarriage journey, I realized God had brought me to this point in my life for a reason. It's my belief that all human beings on earth have a preordained pathway leading toward their highest spiritual potential. There are limitless corridors of possibilities to endeavor on, but choosing the correct path for our own uniquely designed purpose is quite a rare achievement, due to the many challenges one must face to reach that goal. It is dependent on five crucial factors: response to hardship, strategies of survival, willingness to release societal obligations, openness to experiences of the unknown, and the ability to function without definition. If a person's soul is able to conquer these five fundamental trials, they will be light-years ahead of the vast majority of the human race, who spend their entire lives discontent in their bewilderment yet unyielding to change.

I could not change my life, my spirit, my level of happiness, or the outcome of my future. If I continued to be unwilling to learn the deep, resonating spiritual truths from each significant experience in my life, I would have to continue learning them over and over. God gave me an opportunity to heal from my first miscarriage, and in that healing I found peace with my past. Then my second miscarriage helped me to face the unexpected tragic circumstances of life, and because of this, I have begun a much greater journey than any I might have designed for myself. I have started living God's design for my life.

When I finally became willing to come to the Lord to ask him a few questions, my two biggest fears were either he wouldn't answer or I would not like his answer. However, I came to realize that whether or not I liked his answers I couldn't change it either way, and this is how I began to understand the importance of truth and the meaning of faith in my life.

The first major question I wanted to ask God was, *Why?* Just one word, yet it was a loaded question. *Why did this happen to me? Why do you always take the people I love? Why am I not good enough? Why don't you love me? Why don't I belong? Why don't you let me die? Why am I here? Why, why, why?* I couldn't imagine what good could ever come from my loss, but here again God brought me to his Word.

All praise to God, the Father of our Lord Jesus Christ. God is our merciful Father and the source of all comfort. He comforts us in all our troubles so that we can comfort others. When they are troubled, we will be able to give them the same comfort God has given us. For the more we suffer for Christ, the more God will shower us with his comfort through Christ. Even when we are weighed down with troubles, it is for your comfort and salvation! For when we ourselves are comforted, we will certainly comfort you. Then you can patiently endure the same things we suffer. We are confident that as you share in our sufferings, you will also share in the comfort God gives us.

2 Corinthians 1:3–7

I started to realize another purpose in my loss. God was beginning to lead me to share my story with other women and to offer comfort and love, as he provided it for me. I found a scripture in 1 Peter that only continued to reinforce that calling.

Give all your worries and cares to God, for he cares about you. Stay alert! Watch out for your great enemy, the devil. He prowls around like a roaring lion, looking for someone to devour. Stand firm against him, and be strong in your faith. Remember that your Christian brothers and sisters all over the world are going through the same kind of suffering you are. In his kindness God called you to share in his eternal glory by means of Christ Jesus. So after you have suffered a little while, he will restore, support, and strengthen you, and he will place you on a firm foundation. All power to him forever! Amen.

1 Peter 5:7–11

I could finally see that this experience has been for a good purpose. Mothers of miscarriage need a voice, and I am willing to do that. I have been through many trials in my life, but now I have begun to understand what Paul meant in Philippians.

> I know how to live on almost nothing or with everything. I have learned the secret of living in every situation, whether it is with a full stomach or empty, with plenty or little. For I can do everything through Christ, who gives me strength.
>
> Philippians 4:12–13

The secret to surviving my miscarriage was in prayer, studying God's Word, and reaching out to others who have gone through the same sorrows. Of course, it would never have done any good if I had not faced this journey with honesty. Honesty with myself, especially. I felt like everyone was sending me secret messages that forbade me to grieve, but I needed to give *myself* permission to grieve in my own way and in my own time. I did not grieve for Elizabeth until four years after her loss. I did not grieve for my parents for many years and didn't truly seek God's healing for even more years! Time did not heal all my wounds. *God* healed them.

My strategy to survive this nightmare was to learn from it and to give it a purpose. I realized that the majority of the blockades between God and me were within my own mind, and I had to become willing to remove those blockades at whatever cost. I would need to lay down new boundaries. When I heard Jesus' words from Matthew 5:30, "If your hand … causes you to sin, cut it off and throw it away. It is better for you to lose one part of your body than for your whole body to be thrown into hell," I knew that he was calling me to remove from my spiritual body any negatives that hindered me from fully coming to God.

Once I removed the blockades between God and myself, I was able to move on to the next step without any hindrances. This step was openness. Being open-minded to what God could do, in spite of what others define as impossible, is not an easy task. Nevertheless, I was so devastated by my tragedy that I was willing to see, hear, feel, and live life in any new way, even if it was outside the norm. Anything seemed better than the state of mind I was in. So I started looking and listening for God in unconventional ways.

One of the most comforting ways is also one of the most controversial for those who have not experienced it themselves. These are moments that I call "whispers from heaven." It's not only a quiet, still voice that brings peace; it's also a voice defined by association. It's when I walk into the kitchen and get a scent of my mother after all these years of her being gone. It's when I see her favorite butterfly, and she comes immediately to my mind. It's also when I feel a sudden burst of breathtaking wind that I am reminded that my Sammi loves me. Every time I see someone running by out the corner of my eye and no one is there, I remember my Elizabeth. God uses all sorts of ways to remind me of those that I love and have lost.

One windy Sunday morning, nearly two months after we buried our Samantha, we had an amazing whisper from heaven. As we walked toward church, Allie ran ahead of us. A sudden leaf-filled tornado of wind swirled specifically around her. She laughed and ran back to us. Immediately, I thought of my two girls. I could picture their little spirits holding hands and spinning a circle around Allie, laughing and playing. Jack said, "What do you think Sammi and Elizabeth are doing?"

I gasped and said, "I was just thinking that! I thought, *They are playing ring-around-the-rosy!*" It takes only these small occasions for us to appreciate how God allows us to link together with our loved ones in a moment of undefined, certainly irrational by scientific standards, spiritual connection. I know it seems crazy to those who ignore their whispers, but for my own comfort, I choose to listen. I choose to know that God is infinitely more powerful and creative than I could ever limit him to be. I choose to be open to any way he wishes to teach me, even if no one on the planet can understand or define it. It is part of what I call faith!

> Faith is the confidence that what we hope for will actually happen; it gives us assurance about things we cannot see. By faith we understand that the entire universe was formed at God's command, that what we now see did not come from anything that can be seen.
>
> Hebrews 11:1, 3

The most critical part of my healing has been acceptance, another aspect of faith. It's the part of faith that defines trust. The hardest part about this lesson was accepting myself. I have lived my entire life trying to be what others wanted me to be, and finally it occurred to me, *You will never be what others want because they don't know what they really want, and neither do you! It's always changing.* I realized that I was not only allowing

Satan to feed me negative images of my old memories, but he was also defining my negative opinions about myself. Being so critical of myself had led to me being critical of those around me. But God's love abounds in acceptance of who I am. My lack of acceptance of my life was *not* from God. I needed to accept myself, my life, and my circumstances for what they are at present while seeking his will. I had to accept that God knows what he is doing and that each moment is leading up to a bigger moment that I cannot always foresee. This is where faith and acceptance equaled me trusting God.

As I look over my years thus far, I recognize that I am being trained. I am being fashioned as a soldier of the Lord to be the most effective spirit I can be. Each moment and experience in and of itself can mean nothing, but utilized and combined, each leads to another more deepening experience. My objective is to keep my focus on the immediate situation without losing my ability to see the overall picture. If I focus on just one hardship and dismiss the overall picture, I easily get lost in my momentary circumstances. On the other hand, if I concentrate entirely on the larger picture, I risk losing the opportunity to gain the knowledge and growth needed from that specific moment that is meant to aid me in surviving the next hardship.

My journey has not been meaningless, though Satan would have me believe that. Each hardship left a gaping hole in my heart. Those holes *had* to be filled, whether I liked it or not. But if I didn't choose to fill them with God and his truth, then Satan would begin to automatically fill them with lies leading to my feelings of separation from God. By filling these holes with truth, I was benefiting my own soul and my ever-expanding relationship with God.

Jesus replied, "'You must love the Lord your God with all your heart, all your soul, and all your mind.' This is the first and greatest commandment. A second is equally important: 'Love your neighbor as yourself.' The entire law and all the demands of the prophets are based on these two commandments."

Matthew 22:37–40

I try every day to put my beliefs into practice as Paul teaches in his letter to the Philippians:

Always be full of joy in the Lord. I say it again—rejoice! Let everyone see that you are considerate in all you do. Remember, the Lord is coming soon. Don't worry about anything; instead, pray about everything. Tell God what you need, and thank him for all he has done. Then you will experience God's peace, which exceeds anything we can understand. His peace will guard your hearts and minds as you live in Christ Jesus. And now, dear brothers and sisters, one final thing. Fix your thoughts on what is true, and honorable, and right, and pure, and lovely, and admirable. Think about things that are excellent and worthy of praise. Keep putting into practice all you learned and received from me—everything you heard from me and saw me doing. Then the God of peace will be with you.

Philippians 4:4–9

This is my prayer for the mothers of babies born to heaven:

> Lord, I thank you for your wisdom. I thank you for your love. I understand the hurt and sorrow of miscarriage, and I pray that each mother who has lost a baby in any way would read these words and know that you are God. I pray that you would guide their hearts to freedom through your Word and that their journey of sorrow would not end in sorrow but would continue on to your desired destination of healing, trust in you, and love. I pray this in Jesus' holy name, amen.